医学英语新医科课程群系列教材

公共医学英语教程

English for General Medical Purposes

主　编　王长友　延边大学外国语学院
　　　　周宪春　延边大学附属医院（延边医院）
副主编　栾新华　延边大学外国语学院
　　　　崔银峰　延边大学医学院
　　　　全　薇　延边大学外国语学院
　　　　李红英　延边大学外国语学院
　　　　王海洋　天津工业大学生命科学学院
编　委　赵丽丽　延边大学附属医院（延边医院）
　　　　余宁宁　延边大学外国语学院
　　　　张默函　延边大学医学院
　　　　郭书法　蚌埠医学院
　　　　黄　芳　哈尔滨医科大学
　　　　景　然　中国医科大学

U0360296

 南京大学出版社

图书在版编目(CIP)数据

公共医学英语教程 / 王长友,周宪春主编. -- 南京:
南京大学出版社,2022.9
ISBN 978 - 7 - 305 - 26004 - 9

Ⅰ. ①公… Ⅱ. ①王… ②周… Ⅲ. ①医学－英语－
教材 Ⅳ. ①R

中国版本图书馆 CIP 数据核字(2022)第 135894 号

出版发行　南京大学出版社
社　　址　南京市汉口路 22 号　　　　　邮　编　210093
出 版 人　金鑫荣
书　　名　**公共医学英语教程**
主　　编　王长友　周宪春
责任编辑　裴维维　　　　　　　　编辑热线　025 - 83592123
照　　排　南京南琳图文制作有限公司
印　　刷　南京人民印刷厂有限责任公司
开　　本　787×1092　1/16　印张 16.25　字数 450 千
版　　次　2022 年 9 月第 1 版　2022 年 9 月第 1 次印刷
ISBN 978 - 7 - 305 - 26004 - 9
定　　价　49.00 元

网址:http://www.njupco.com
官方微博:http://weibo.com/njupco
官方微信号:njupress
销售咨询热线:(025) 83594756

前　言

《国家中长期教育改革和发展规划纲要(2010—2020 年)》《关于加快建设高水平本科教育全面提高人才培养能力的意见》和《关于加强医教协同实施卓越医生教育培养计划 2.0 的意见》等都提出培养复合型和国际化人才的要求。在新医科背景下,本教材基于《大学英语教学指南》(2020 版)对 ESP 教学的要求而编写。

教材共分 10 个单元,以人体系统的常见疾病为线索进行编排:每个单元分别选取不同人体系统的 4 种常见疾病(每种疾病约 1100 字),按病因、症状、诊断、治疗等框架展开,每单元的 Text A 和 Text B 是主课文,文后附有翻译、口语和实用医学英语写作等练习;每单元的 Text C 和 Text D 是副课文,文后附有相关医学词汇,可根据课时情况作为补充阅读。

全书材料选自相关医学网站和国内相关书籍,由从事医学专业教学的西医教师、从事语言教学的英语教育教师和从事医学英语教学的医学英语教师精选、审稿、汇编而成,保证了语言表达的地道性和医学内容的准确性。

本教材与其他同类教材相比,其特点是系统性、针对性、实用性和时代性。

1. 系统性。教材以人体系统为基本编排框架,有效地将医学各科内容串联起来。

2. 针对性。本教材根据地方性医学院校学生的英语水平编写,语言地道易懂,适合作为从 EGP 到 EMP 的过渡教材,能有效引导学生顺利进入医学英语的学习。

3. 实用性。教材内容涉及医学各科,涵盖医学生在未来职业生涯中所常接触的素材,实用性较强。

4. 时代性。教材紧跟时代前沿,热点文章将在二维码平台更新,供读者参考、学习。

王长友、栾新华、全薇、李红英负责教材语言层面的校对,周宪春、崔银峰负责教材医学专业内容的校对。具体分工如下:王长友负责本书的总体策划、编写分工、体例制订、统稿、每单元 Text A 和 Text B 的词汇提取和练习的编写。各单元英语版疾病及视频资料的查找和节选:周宪春负责 Units 1—5,崔银峰负责 Units 6—9,栾新华负责 Unit 10 及二维码中拓展阅读内容的更新。副课文医学词汇的提取:栾新华负责 Units 1—3,全薇负责 Units 4—6,李红英负责 Units 7—10。电子信息专业硕士研究生王海洋负责教材配套视频资料的剪辑和文字提取(共 20 个),美籍外教 Robert Tench 对视频的文字进行了校对。其他编委负责自己分工的任务。

本教材的编写得到延边大学医学院及附属医院、蚌埠医学院、中国医科大学、哈尔滨医科大学等专家教师的大力支持和帮助。出版社对教材的编写和出版做了大量的工作，在此谨致以真诚的感谢！

由于我们水平有限，教材难免存在不当和谬误之处，恳请广大读者批评指正，以便我们对本教材进行修订。

本教材是吉林省"十四五"规划2021年度重点课题（ZD21021）成果之一。

编委会

2022 年 6 月

CONTENTS

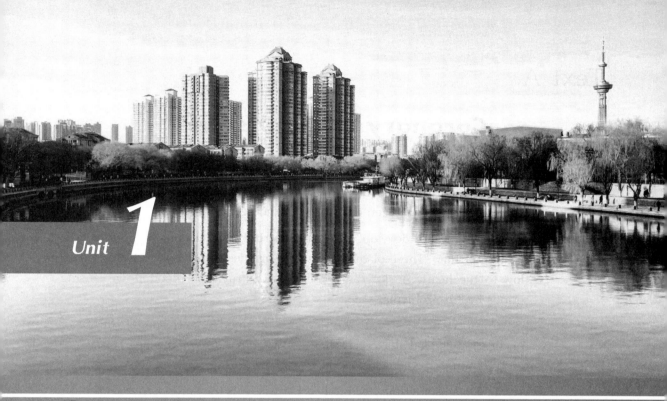

Unit **1**

Some Common Diseases of the Circulatory System

✓参考答案
✓微课等资源

Text A

Coronary Heart Disease

Coronary heart disease (CHD), or coronary artery disease, develops when the coronary arteries become too narrow. The coronary arteries are the blood vessels that supply oxygen and blood to the heart.

CHD tends to develop when cholesterol builds up on the artery walls, creating **plaques**. These plaques cause the arteries to narrow, reducing blood flow to the heart. A clot can sometimes obstruct the blood flow, causing serious health problems.

Coronary arteries form the network of blood vessels on the surface of the heart that feed it oxygen. If these arteries narrow, the heart may not receive enough oxygen-rich blood, especially during physical activity.

CHD can sometimes lead to heart attack. It is the "most common type of heart disease in the United States", where it accounts for more than 370,000 deaths every year.

Causes

CHD develops as a result of injury or damage to the inner layer of a coronary artery. This damage causes fatty deposits of plaque to build up at the injury site. These deposits consist of cholesterol and other waste products from cells. This buildup is called **atherosclerosis**.

If pieces of plaque break off or **rupture**, platelets will **cluster** in the area in an attempt to repair the blood vessel. This cluster can block the artery and reduce or block blood flow, which may lead to a heart attack.

Symptoms

CHD can lead to **angina**. This is a type of chest pain linked to heart disease. Angina may cause the following feelings across the chest:

- Squeezing;
- Pressure;
- Heaviness;
- Tightening;
- Burning;

- Aching.

Angina might also cause the following symptoms:

- Indigestion;
- Heartburn;
- Weakness;
- Sweating;
- **Nausea**;
- **Cramping**.

CHD can also lead to shortness of breath. If the heart and other organs do not receive enough oxygen, any form of exertion can become very tiring, which may cause a person to **pant** for air.

Risk factors

The following factors increase a person's risk of developing CHD:

- Having high blood pressure, or hypertension;
- Having high levels of low-density lipoprotein, or "bad" cholesterol;
- Having low levels of high-density lipoprotein, or "good" cholesterol;
- Having a diagnosis of diabetes, in which the body cannot effectively remove sugar from the bloodstream;
- Having obesity;
- Smoking, which increases inflammation and increases cholesterol deposits in the coronary arteries.

Some risk factors are not lifestyle-related. These may include:

- Having high levels of the amino acid **homocysteine**, which one 2015 study linked to a higher incidence of CHD;
- Having high levels of **fibrinogen**, a blood protein that encourages the clumping of platelets to form blood clots;
- Having a family history of CHD;
- For women, having been through menopause;
- For men, being over 45 years of age.

Having high levels of lipoprotein(a) specifically is also linked to a higher risk of cardiovascular disease and CHD.

Diagnosis

A doctor can perform a physical examination, and order a number of tests to diagnose CHD. For example:

- **Electrocardiogram**: This records the electrical activity and rhythm of the heart.
- **Holter monitor**: This is a portable device that a person wears under their clothes for 2 days or more. It records all the electrical activity of the heart, including the heartbeat.
- **Echocardiogram**: This is an ultrasound scan that monitors the pumping heart. It uses sound waves to provide a video image.
- Stress test: This may involve the use of a **treadmill** or medication that stresses the heart in order to test how it functions when a person is active.
- Coronary **catheterization**: A specialist will inject dye through a **catheter** which they have **threaded** through an artery, often in the leg or arm. The dye shows narrow spots or blockages on an X-ray.
- CT scans: These help the doctor visualize the arteries, detect calcium within fatty deposits, and characterize any heart **anomalies**.
- Nuclear **ventriculography**: This uses tracers, or radioactive materials, to create an image of the heart chambers. A doctor will inject the tracers into the vein. The tracers then attach to red blood cells and pass through the heart. Special cameras or scanners trace the movement of the tracers.
- Blood tests: Doctors can run these to measure blood cholesterol levels, especially in people at risk of high blood cholesterol levels.

Treatment

There is no cure for CHD. However, there are ways that a person can manage the condition. Treatment tends to involve making healthful lifestyle changes, such as quitting smoking, adopting a healthful diet, and getting regular exercise. However, some people may need to take medications or undergo medical procedures.

Medications

Medications that people can take to reduce the risk or impact of CHD include:

- Beta-blockers: A doctor may prescribe beta-blockers to reduce blood pressure and heart rate, especially among people who have already had a heart attack.
- **Nitroglycerin** patches, sprays, or tablets: These relax the arteries and reduce the heart's demand for blood, as well as soothe chest pain.
- **Angiotensin**-converting enzyme inhibitors: These bring down blood pressure and help slow or stop the progression of CHD.
- Calcium channel blockers: These will widen the coronary arteries,

improving blood flow to the heart and reducing hypertension.

• **Statins**: These may have a positive impact on outcomes in CHD. One 2019 review found that although taking statins cannot reduce the overall risk of death from CHD, they can prevent development and reduce the risk of non-fatal heart attacks. However, they might not be effective for people with cholesterol disorders such as **hyperlipidemia**.

In the past, some people used aspirin to lower their risk of CHD, but current guidelines only recommend this for people with a high risk of heart attack, stroke, angina, or other cardiovascular events. This is because aspirin is a blood thinner, which increases a person's risk of bleeding. Doctors now recommend focusing on lifestyle strategies, such as adopting a healthful diet and getting regular moderate to intense exercise. These strategies can reduce the risk of atherosclerosis.

Surgery

The following surgical procedures can open or replace blocked arteries if they have become very narrow, or if symptoms are not responding to medications:

• Laser surgery: This involves making several very small holes in the heart muscle. These encourage the formation of new blood vessels.

• Coronary **bypass** surgery: A surgeon will use a blood vessel from another part of the body to create a **graft** that bypasses the blocked artery. The graft may come from the leg, for example, or an inner chest wall artery.

• **Angioplasty** and stent placement: A surgeon will insert a catheter into the narrowed part of the artery and pass a **deflated** balloon through the catheter to the affected area. When they **inflate** the balloon, it compresses the fatty deposits against the artery walls. They may leave a **stent**, or mesh tube, in the artery to help keep it open.

On rare occasions, a person may need a heart transplant. However, this is only if the heart has severe damage and treatment is not working.

(1186 words)

◆ **Vocabulary**

coronary [ˈkɒrənri] *adj.* 冠的，冠状的，冠状动脉的

coronary heart disease 冠心病

plaque [plæk; plɑːk] *n.* 斑（块）；匾

atherosclerosis [ˌæθərəʊsklɪəˈrəʊsɪs] *n.* [内科] 动脉粥样硬化，动脉硬化

rupture [ˈrʌptʃə(r)] n. 破裂，决裂；疝气 vi. 破裂；发疝气

cluster [ˈklʌstə(r)] vt. 使聚集 vi. 群聚，丛生 n. 群，簇，丛，串

angina [ænˈdʒaɪnə] n. 心绞痛

nausea [ˈnɔːziə] n. 恶心，晕船

cramp [ˈkræmp] n. 肌肉一时局部麻痹，(痛性)痉挛

pant [pænt] v. 渴望；气喘，喘息

homocysteine [həʊməˈsɪstiːn] n. [生化] 同型半胱氨酸，高半胱氨酸，巯基丁氨酸

fibrinogen [faɪˈbrɪnədʒən] n. [生化] 血纤蛋白原；纤维蛋白原

electrocardiogram [ɪˌlektrəʊˈkɑːdiəʊɡræm] n. [内科] 心电图

Holter monitor 霍尔特氏心电动态监测仪；动态心电图监护仪

echocardiogram [ˌekəʊˈkɑːdiəʊɡræm] n. [内科] 超声心动图，心回波图

treadmill [ˈtredmɪl] n. 踏车，跑步机

catheterization [ˈkæθɪtəˌraɪzeɪʃən] n. [外科] 导管插入

catheter [ˈkæθətə(r)] n. [医] 导管，导尿管，尿液管

thread [θred] vt. 穿过，穿(针) n. 线

anomaly [əˈnɒməli] n. 异常，不规则，反常事物

ventriculography [venˌtrɪkjʊˈlɒɡrəfi] n. [特医] 心室造影术，脑室造影术

nitroglycerin [ˌnaɪtrəʊˈɡlɪsəriːn] n. 硝酸甘油，硝化甘油，甘油三硝酸酯

angiotensin [ˌændʒɪəʊˈtensən] n. 血管紧张肽，血管紧缩素

statin [ˈstætɪn] n. 他汀类，抑制素

hyperlipidemia [ˌhaɪpəˌlɪpɪˈdiːmiə] n. 高脂血，血脂过多

bypass [ˈbaɪpɑːs] n. 旁路，支路，旁通管；分流术 v. 绕过，避开

graft [ɡrɑːft] n. 嫁接，移植

angioplasty [ˈændʒɪəˌplæsti] n. 血管成形术

deflate [dɪˈfleɪt] vt. 放气，使缩小

inflate [ɪnˈfleɪt] vt. 使充气，使通货膨胀 vi. 膨胀，充气

stent [stent] n. 支架

◆ **Exercises** ◆

Ⅰ. **Decide whether the following sentences are *True* or *False* according to the text.**

1. The coronary arteries are the blood vessels that supply oxygen and blood to the heart and brain.

2. When cholesterol builds up on the coronary artery walls and forms plaques, CHD may develop.

3. If pieces of plaque break off from the artery walls, platelets will cluster in the area to repair the blood vessel.

4. Sometimes CHD can lead to heart attack, but can't lead to angina.

5. The symptoms of weakness, nausea and heartburn might be caused by angina.

6. Low levels of high-density lipoprotein is "good" cholesterol, but high levels of low-density lipoprotein is "bad" cholesterol.

7. The risk factors of developing CHD include smoking, having hypertension, etc.

8. Electrocardiogram can help the doctors to diagnose CHD, but blood test is excluded.

9. Medications, surgery and healthful lifestyle changes can cure CHD.

10. Calcium channel blockers can widen the coronary arteries and improve blood flow to the heart.

Ⅱ. **Fill in the blanks with the proper form of words in the box.**

thrombosis	hyperlipidemia	angiotensin	atherosclerosis	angina
clammy	catheter	cramp	angioplasty	ventriculography

1. _____ is the build up of a waxy plaque on the inside of blood vessels. In Greek, *athere* means gruel, and *skleros* means hard.

2. _____ is chest pain or pressure, usually due to not enough blood flow to the heart muscle.

3. _____ is a painful involuntary muscle spasm, which may result from loss of salt owing to excessive sweating or from deficient blood supply to the affected area.

4. _____ is the formation of a blood clot inside a blood vessel, obstructing the flow of blood through the circulatory system.

5. His skin felt cold and _____ , so he put on his overcoat to prevent cold.

6. _____ is a peptide hormone that causes vasoconstriction and an increase in blood pressure.

7. _____ is abnormally elevated levels of any or all lipids or lipoproteins in the blood.

8. _____ is a minimally invasive endovascular procedure used to widen narrowed or obstructed arteries or veins, typically to treat arterial atherosclerosis.

9. _____ is a thin tube made from medical grade materials serving a broad range of functions.

10. _____ is of great value in locating the tumor.

Ⅲ. **Translation: translate the passage into Chinese.**

There are two main causes of stroke: a blocked artery (ischemic stroke) or leaking or bursting of a blood vessel (hemorrhagic stroke). Some people may have only a temporary disruption of blood flow to the brain, known as a transient ischemic attack (TIA), that doesn't cause lasting symptoms.

Ischemic stroke is the most common type of stroke. It happens when the brain's blood vessels become narrowed or blocked, causing severely reduced blood flow (ischemia). Blocked or narrowed blood vessels are caused by fatty deposits that build up in blood vessels or by blood clots or other debris that travel through your bloodstream and lodge in the blood vessels in your brain. Some initial research shows that COVID-19 infection may be a possible cause of ischemic stroke, but more study is needed.

Hemorrhagic stroke occurs when a blood vessel in your brain leaks or ruptures. Brain hemorrhages can result from many conditions that affect your blood vessels. Factors related to hemorrhagic stroke include: uncontrolled high blood pressure, bulges at weak spots in your blood vessel walls (aneurysms), trauma, protein deposits in blood vessel walls that lead to weakness in the vessel wall, ischemic stroke leading to hemorrhage. A less common cause of bleeding in the brain is arteriovenous malformation.

A transient ischemic attack (TIA)—sometimes known as a ministroke—is a temporary period of symptoms similar to those you'd have in a stroke. A TIA doesn't cause permanent damage. They're caused by a temporary decrease in blood supply to part of your brain, which may last as little as five minutes. Like an ischemic stroke, a TIA occurs when a clot or debris reduces or blocks blood flow to part of your nervous system. Seek emergency care even if you think you've had a TIA. It's not possible to tell if you're having a stroke or TIA based only on your symptoms. If you've had a TIA, it means you may have a partially blocked or narrowed artery leading to your brain. Having a TIA increases your risk of having a full-blown stroke later.

（344 words）

Ⅳ. **Give a presentation.**

Dictate the causes, symptoms, treatments, etc. of Coronary Heart Disease in English with 3—4 students. Try to use the formal expression, especially related medical terminology when you make your presentation.

Ⅴ. **Write a letter of application.**

请根据下列内容写封留学申请信：

我已于 2020 年获得同济大学医学院的学士学位，想申请到耶鲁大学临床医学专业攻读硕士学位，拟定于 2023 年秋天入学。如可能，希望能获得研究生助教奖学金。我的地址：上海市长宁区东西路 34 号 205 室，200003。

Text B

High Blood Pressure

High blood pressure (**hypertension**) is a common condition in which the long-term force of the blood against your artery walls is high enough that it may eventually cause health problems, such as heart disease. Blood pressure is determined both by the amount of blood your heart pumps and the amount of resistance to blood flow in your arteries. The more blood your heart pumps and the narrower your arteries, the higher your blood pressure. A blood pressure reading is given in millimeters of mercury (mm Hg). It has two numbers.

- Top number (**systolic** pressure). The first, or upper, number measures the pressure in your arteries when your heart beats.
- Bottom number (**diastolic** pressure). The second, or lower, number measures the pressure in your arteries between beats.

You can have high blood pressure for years without any symptoms. Uncontrolled high blood pressure increases your risk of serious health problems, including heart attack and stroke. Fortunately, high blood pressure can be easily detected. And once you know you have high blood pressure, you can work with your doctor to control it.

Symptoms

Most people with high blood pressure have no signs or symptoms, even if blood pressure readings reach dangerously high levels.

A few people with high blood pressure may have headaches, shortness of breath or nosebleeds, but these signs and symptoms aren't specific and usually don't occur until high blood pressure has reached a severe or life-threatening stage.

Causes

There are two types of high blood pressure.

Primary (essential) hypertension

For most adults, there's no identifiable cause of high blood pressure. This type of high blood pressure, called primary (essential) hypertension, tends to develop gradually over many years.

Secondary hypertension

Some people have high blood pressure caused by an underlying condition. This type of high blood pressure, called secondary hypertension, tends to appear suddenly and cause higher blood pressure than does primary hypertension. Various conditions and medications can lead to secondary hypertension, including:

- **Obstructive sleep apnea**;
- Kidney disease;
- Adrenal gland tumors;
- Thyroid problems;
- Certain defects you're born with (**congenital**) in blood vessels;
- Certain medications, such as birth control pills, cold remedies, **decongestants**, over-the-counter pain relievers and some prescription drugs;
- Illegal drugs, such as cocaine and amphetamines.

Diagnosis

Your doctor will ask questions about your medical history and do a physical examination. The doctor, nurse or other medical assistant will place an inflatable arm cuff around your arm and measure your blood pressure using a pressure-measuring **gauge**. Your blood pressure generally should be measured in both arms to determine if there is a difference. It's important to use an appropriate-sized arm cuff. Blood pressure measurements fall into several categories:

- Normal blood pressure. Your blood pressure is normal if it's below 120/80 mm Hg.
- Elevated blood pressure. Elevated blood pressure is a systolic pressure ranging from 120 to 139 mm Hg and (or) a diastolic pressure ranging from 80 to 89 mm Hg. Elevated blood pressure tends to get worse over time unless steps are taken to control blood pressure. Elevated blood pressure may also be called prehypertension.
- Stage 1 hypertension. Stage 1 hypertension is a systolic pressure ranging from 140 to 159 mm Hg and (or) a diastolic pressure ranging from 90 to 99 mm Hg.
- Stage 2 hypertension. Stage 2 hypertension is a systolic pressure ranging from 160 to 179 mm Hg and (or) a diastolic pressure ranging from 100 to 109 mm Hg.
- Stage 3 hypertension. Stage 3 hypertension is a systolic pressure of

180 mm Hg or higher and (or) a diastolic pressure of 110 mm Hg or higher.

• Hypertensive crisis. A blood pressure measurement higher than 180/120 mm Hg is an emergency situation that requires urgent medical care.

Tests

If you have high blood pressure, your doctor may recommend tests to confirm the diagnosis and check for underlying conditions that can cause hypertension.

• **Ambulatory** monitoring. This 24-hour blood pressure monitoring test is used to confirm if you have high blood pressure.

• Lab tests. Your doctor may recommend a urine test (**urinalysis**) and blood tests, including a cholesterol test.

• Electrocardiogram (ECG or EKG). This quick and painless test measures your heart's electrical activity.

• Echocardiogram. Depending on your signs and symptoms and test results, your doctor may order an echocardiogram to check for more signs of heart disease. An echocardiogram uses sound waves to produce images of the heart.

Treatment

Changing your lifestyle can help control and manage high blood pressure. Your doctor may recommend that you make lifestyle changes including:

• Eating a heart-healthy diet with less salt;
• Getting regular physical activity;
• Maintaining a healthy weight or losing weight if you're overweight or obese;
• Limiting the amount of alcohol you drink.

But sometimes lifestyle changes aren't enough. If diet and exercise don't help, your doctor may recommend medication to lower your blood pressure.

Medications

The type of medication your doctor prescribes for high blood pressure depends on your blood pressure measurements and overall health. Two or more blood pressure drugs often work better than one. Medications used to treat high blood pressure include:

• **Diuretics**. Diuretics, sometimes called water pills, are medications that help your kidneys eliminate sodium and water from the body. These drugs are often the first medications tried to treat high blood pressure.

• Angiotensin-converting enzyme (ACE) inhibitors. These medications—

such as **lisinopril**, **benazepril**, **captopril** and others—help relax blood vessels by blocking the formation of a natural chemical that narrows blood vessels.

• Angiotensin Ⅱ **receptor blockers** (ARBs). These medications relax blood vessels by blocking the action, not the formation, of a natural chemical that narrows blood vessels. ARBs include **candesartan**, losartan and others.

• Calcium channel blockers. These medications—including **amlodipine**, **diltiazem** and others—help relax the muscles of your blood vessels.

Additional medications sometimes used to treat high blood pressure

If you're having trouble reaching your blood pressure goal with combinations of the above medications, your doctor may prescribe:

• Alpha blockers. These medications reduce nerve signals to blood vessels, lowering the effects of natural chemicals that narrow blood vessels.

• Alpha-beta blockers. Alpha-beta blockers block nerve signals to blood vessels and slow the heartbeat to reduce the amount of blood that must be pumped through the vessels.

• Beta blockers. These medications reduce the workload on your heart and widen your blood vessels, causing your heart to beat slower and with less force.

• **Aldosterone antagonists**. These drugs also are considered diuretics. These drugs block the effect of a natural chemical that can lead to salt and fluid buildup, which can contribute to high blood pressure. They may be used to treat resistant hypertension.

• **Renin** inhibitors. **Aliskiren** (Tekturna) slows the production of renin, an enzyme produced by your kidneys that starts a chain of chemical steps that increases blood pressure.

• **Vasodilators**. These medications work directly on the muscles in the walls of your arteries, preventing the muscles from tightening and your arteries from narrowing.

• Central-acting agents. These medications prevent your brain from telling your nervous system to increase your heart rate and narrow your blood vessels.

You should always take blood pressure medications as prescribed. Never skip a dose or abruptly stop taking your blood pressure medication. Suddenly stopping certain blood pressure drugs, such as beta blockers, can cause a sharp increase in blood pressure (rebound hypertension).

(1237 words)

Vocabulary

hypertension [ˌhaɪpəˈtenʃn] *n.* 高血压；过度紧张

systolic [ˌsɪsˈtɒlɪk] *adj.* 心脏收缩的

diastolic [ˌdaɪəˈstɒlɪk] *adj.* 心脏舒张的

apnea [ˈæpnɪə] *n.* [医] 窒息，[临床] 呼吸暂停

obstructive sleep apnea [内科] 阻塞性睡眠呼吸暂停

congenital [kənˈdʒenɪtl] *adj.* 先天的，天生的；天赋的

decongestant [ˌdi:kənˈdʒestənt] *n.* 减充血药

gauge [geɪdʒ] *n.* 计量器，标准尺寸，容量规格

ambulatory [ˈæmbjələtəri] *adj.* 流动的，走动的，非固定的

urinalysis [ˌjʊərɪˈnælɪsɪs] *n.* 尿分析

diuretic [ˌdaɪjʊˈretɪk] *n.* [药] 利尿剂 *adj.* 利尿的

lisinopril [lɪzɪˈnəʊprɪl] *n.* 赖诺普利（一种抑制剂）

benazepril *n.* 苯那普利

captopril [ˈkæpˈtɒprɪl] *n.* 甲巯丙脯酸

receptor blocker 受体阻断剂

candesartan *n.* 坎地沙坦

amlodipine [æmˈləʊdɪpɪn] *n.* 氨氯地平（抗高血压药）

diltiazem [daɪˈtaɪəˌzem] *n.* 地尔硫卓（一种新型的钙离子拮抗剂）

aldosterone [ælˈdɒstərəʊn] *n.* 醛甾酮

antagonist [ænˈtæɡənɪst] *n.* [医] 对抗剂

renin [ˈriːnɪn] *n.* [生化] 肾素，高血压蛋白原酶

aliskiren 阿利吉仑(第二代肾素抑制剂)

vasodilator [ˌveɪzəʊdaɪˈleɪtə] *n.* [药] [生理] 血管舒张药，血管扩张神经

Exercises

I. **Decide whether the following sentences are *True* or *False* according to the text.**

1. High blood pressure refers to the long-term force of the blood against the venous walls.

2. Diastolic pressure refers to the pressure in your arteries when your heart beats.

3. Most people with high blood pressure will have some signs or symptoms.

4. Two types of high blood pressure include primary and secondary hypertension.

5. Essential hypertension means there are identifiable causes of high blood pressure.

6. Kidney disease, thyroid problems and illegal drugs can lead to secondary hypertension.

7. Prehypertension means a systolic pressure ranges from 140 to 159 mm Hg.

8. Electrocardiogram can measure your heart's electrical activity.

9. Lifestyle changes can help control hypertension, but medications can cure it.

10. People with hypertension should always take blood pressure medications, without abruptly stopping taking it.

Ⅱ. Fill in the blanks with the proper form of words in the box.

| atherosclerosis | apnea | diastolic | echocardiogram | systolic |
| hypertension | urinalysis | thyroid | aneurysm | dementia |

1. _____ is elevated blood pressure resulting from an increase in the amount of blood.

2. A _____ blood pressure reading below 120 is considered normal.

3. When your blood pressure is measured, there are two readings: systolic and _____.

4. _____ is cessation of breathing, especially during sleep.

5. Located near the base of the neck, the _____ is a large endocrine gland that produces hormones that help control growth and metabolism.

6. _____ is a disease in which the wall of the artery develops abnormalities, called lesions.

7. _____ is localized dilatation of a blood vessel, particularly an artery, or the heart.

8. _____ is a loss of mental ability severe enough to interfere with normal activities of daily living.

9. _____ is a diagnostic physical, chemical, and microscopic examination of a urine sample.

10. _____ is a non-invasive ultrasound test that shows an image of the inside of the heart.

Ⅲ. Translation: translate the passage into Chinese.

How High Blood Pressure Can Lead to Stroke

Stroke and high blood pressure

Stroke is a leading cause of death and severe, long-term disability. Most people who've had a first stroke also had high blood pressure (HBP or hypertension).

High blood pressure damages arteries throughout the body, creating conditions where they can burst or clog more easily. Weakened arteries in the brain, resulting from high blood pressure, put you at a much higher risk for stroke, which is why managing high blood pressure is critical to reduce your chance of having a stroke.

What happens when you have a stroke

A stroke occurs when a blood vessel to the brain is either blocked by a clot (ischemic stroke) or bursts (hemorrhagic stroke). When that happens, part of the brain is no longer getting the blood and oxygen it needs, so it starts to die. Your brain controls your movement and thoughts, so a stroke doesn't only hurt your brain—it can threaten your ability to think, move and function. Strokes can affect language, memory and vision. Severe strokes may even cause paralysis or death.

A majority of strokes are ischemic strokes—caused by narrowed or clogged blood vessels (atherosclerosis) in the brain that cut off the blood flow to brain cells. A much smaller percentage of strokes are hemorrhagic strokes (cerebral hemorrhages) that occur when a blood vessel ruptures in or near the brain, resulting in a subarachnoid hemorrhage (SAH) on the surface of the brain or intracerebral hemorrhage (ICH) deep within the brain.

ATIA (transient ischemic attack) is caused by a temporary clot. Often called a "mini stroke", these warning strokes should be taken very seriously. Don't let high blood pressure lead to stroke:

- Spot the warning signs of a stroke—FAST!
- Download a fact sheet about how high blood pressure leads to stroke.
- Know your blood pressure numbers.
- Make changes that matter to help prevent stroke.
- Learn the important connection between BP, atrial fibrillation and stroke.

（344 words）

Ⅳ. Give a presentation.

Dictate the causes, symptoms, treatments, etc. of High Blood Pressure in English with 3—4 students. Try to use the formal expression when you make your presentation.

Ⅴ. Write a resume for studying abroad.

根据下列内容,撰写一份个人简历。

李阳,男,1998 年 3 月出生于广东省汕头市,邮箱:liyang@163.com,现地址:中国广州外环东路 280 号,510006。

目的:申请攻读哈佛大学医学院医学硕士学位。

教育:2017 年 9 月至今在复旦大学上海医学院学习。

专业：临床医学专业

主要课程：人体解剖学、组织胚胎学、生理学、生物化学、病理学、诊断学、外科学、内科学、妇产科学、儿科学等。

目前的平均绩点：3.9/4.0。

奖励和荣誉：获一等奖学金 3 次。

语言能力：大学英语六级证书。

兴趣爱好：慢跑、旅游、流行音乐。

Text C

Valvular Heart Disease

Valvular heart disease is when any valve in the heart has damage or is diseased. There are several causes of valve disease. The normal heart has four chambers (right and left **atria**, and right and left **ventricles**) and four valves. The **mitral** valve, also called the **bicuspid** valve, allows blood to flow from the left atrium to the left ventricle. The **tricuspid** valve allows blood to flow from the right atrium to the right ventricle. The **aortic** valve allows blood to flow from the left ventricle to the aorta. The **pulmonary** valve allows blood to flow from the right ventricle to the pulmonary artery. The valves open and close to control or regulate the blood flowing into the heart and then away from the heart. Three of the heart valves are composed of three leaflets or flaps that work together to open and close to allow blood to flow across the opening. The mitral valve only has two leaflets.

Healthy heart valve leaflets are able to fully open and close the valve during the heartbeat, but diseased valves might not fully open and close. Any valve in the heart can become diseased, but the aortic valve is most commonly affected. Diseased valves can become "leaky" where they don't completely close; this is called regurgitation. If this happens, blood leaks back into the chamber that it came from and not enough blood can be pushed forward through the heart. The other common type of heart valve condition happens when the opening of the valve is narrowed and stiff and the valve is not able to open fully when blood is trying to pass through; this is called **stenosis**.

Sometimes the valve may be missing a leaflet—this more commonly involves the aortic valve. If the heart valves are diseased, the heart can't effectively pump blood throughout the body and has to work harder to pump, either while the blood is leaking back into the chamber or against a narrowed opening. This can lead to heart failure, sudden cardiac arrest (when the heart stops beating), and death.

Facts

- About 2.5% of the U.S. population has valvular heart disease, but it is more common in older adults. About 13% of people born before 1943 have valvular heart disease.

- **Rheumatic** heart disease most commonly affects the mitral valve (which has only two leaflets) or the aortic valve, but any valve can be affected, and more than one can be involved.
- Bicuspid aortic valve (having only two leaflets rather than the normal three) happens in about 1% to 2% of the population and is more common among men.
- In 2017, there were 3,046 deaths due to rheumatic valvular heart disease and 24,811 deaths due to non-rheumatic valvular heart disease in the United States.
- Nearly 25,000 deaths in the U.S. each year are due to heart valve disease from causes other than rheumatic disease.
- Valvular heart disease deaths are more commonly due to aortic valve disease.

Causes

There are several causes of valvular heart disease, including congenital conditions (being born with it), infections, degenerative conditions (wearing out with age), and conditions linked to other types of heart disease.

Rheumatic disease can happen after an infection from the bacteria that causes strep throat is not treated with antibiotics. The infection can cause scarring of the heart valve. This is the most common cause of valve disease worldwide, but it is much less common in the United States, where most strep infections are treated early with antibiotics. It is, however, more common in the United States among people born before 1943.

Endocarditis is an infection of the inner lining of the heart caused by a severe infection in the blood. The infection can settle on the heart valves and damage the leaflets. Intravenous drug use can also lead to endocarditis and cause heart valve disease.

Congenital heart valve disease is malformations of the heart valves, such as missing one of its leaflets. The most commonly affected valve with a congenital defect is a bicuspid aortic valve, which has only two leaflets rather than three.

Other types of heart disease:
- Heart failure. Heart failure happens when the heart cannot pump enough blood and oxygen to support other organs in your body.
- Atherosclerosis of the aorta where it attaches to the heart. Atherosclerosis refers to a buildup of plaque on the inside of the blood vessel.

Plaque is made up of fat, calcium, and cholesterol.

- **Thoracic** aortic **aneurysm**, a **bulge** or ballooning where the aorta attaches to the heart.
- High blood pressure.
- A heart attack (also known as myocardial **infarction** or MI), which can damage the muscles that control the opening and closing of the valve.
- Autoimmune disease, such as **lupus**.
- **Marfan syndrome**, a disease of connective tissue that can affect heart valves.
- Exposure to high-dose radiation, which may lead to calcium deposits on the valve.
- The aging process, which can cause calcium deposits to develop on the heart valves, making them stiff or thickened and less efficient with age.

Symptoms

Heart valve disease can develop quickly or over a long period. When valve disease develops more slowly, there may be no symptoms until the condition is quite advanced. When it develops more suddenly, people may experience the following symptoms:

- Shortness of breath;
- Chest pain;
- Fatigue;
- Dizziness or fainting;
- Fever;
- Rapid weight gain;
- Irregular heartbeat.

Diagnosis

The doctor may hear a **heart murmur** (an unusual sound) when listening to your heartbeat. Depending on the location of the murmur, how it sounds, and its rhythm, the doctor may be able to determine which valve is affected and what type of problem it is (regurgitation or stenosis).

A doctor may also use an echocardiography, a test that uses sound waves to create a movie of the valves to see if they are working correctly.

Treatment

If the condition isn't too severe, it might be managed with medicines to treat the symptoms. If the valve is more seriously diseased and causing more severe symptoms, surgery may be recommended. The type of surgery will depend on the valve involved and the cause of the disease. For some conditions, the valve will need to be replaced by either opening the heart during surgery or replacing the valve without having to open the heart during surgery.

(1071 words)

◆ Vocabulary

valvular heart disease 心脏瓣膜病

atria [ˈɑːtriə] n. 心房；前庭；门廊（atrium 的复数）

ventricle [ˈventrɪkl] n. 室，心室，脑室

mitral [ˈmaɪtrəl] adj. 二尖瓣的

bicuspid [baɪˈkʌpɪd] adj. 有两尖头的，双尖的

tricuspid [traɪˈkʌspɪd] n. 三尖瓣　adj. 三尖的

aortic [eɪˈɔːtɪk] adj. 大动脉的

pulmonary [ˈpʌlmənəri] adj. 肺的，肺部的，肺状的

stenosis [stɪˈnəʊsɪs] n. [病理]（器官）狭窄

rheumatic [ruːˈmætɪk] adj. 风湿病的，风湿病引起的　n. 风湿病，风湿病患者

endocarditis [ˌendəʊkɑːˈdaɪtɪs] n. [内科] 心内膜炎

thoracic [θɔːˈræsɪk] adj. [解剖] 胸的，[解剖] 胸廓的

aneurysm [ˈænjəˌrɪzəm] n. [内科] 动脉瘤 (= aneurism)

bulge [bʌldʒ] n. 胀，膨胀；凸出部分　vt. 使膨胀，使凸起

infarction [ɪnˈfɑːkʃn] n. [病理] 梗死形成

lupus [ˈluːpəs] n. [内科][皮肤] 狼疮

marfan syndrome 马方综合征，马凡综合征

murmur [ˈmɜːmə(r)] n. [医] 心区杂音；低语　v. 低语，低声抱怨

heart murmur [临床] 心杂音

Text D

Endocarditis

Endocarditis is a life-threatening inflammation of the inner lining of your heart's chambers and valves (**endocardium**). Endocarditis is usually caused by an infection. Bacteria, fungi or other germs from another part of your body, such as your mouth, spread through your bloodstream and attach to damaged areas in your heart. If it's not treated quickly, endocarditis can damage or destroy your heart valves. Treatment for endocarditis include medications and, sometimes, surgery. People at greatest risk of endocarditis usually have damaged heart valves, artificial heart valves or other heart defects.

Symptoms

Endocarditis may develop slowly or suddenly, depending on what germs are causing the infection and whether you have any underlying heart problems. Signs and symptoms of endocarditis can vary from person to person.

Common signs and symptoms of endocarditis include:

- Aching joints and muscles;
- Chest pain when you breathe;
- Fatigue;
- Flu-like symptoms, such as fever and chills;
- Night sweats;
- Shortness of breath;
- Swelling in your feet, legs or abdomen;
- A new or changed heart murmur, which is the heart sound made by blood rushing through your heart.

Less common signs and symptoms of endocarditis can include:

- Unexplained weight loss;
- Blood in your urine, which you might be able to see or that your doctor might see when he or she views your urine under a microscope;
- Tenderness in your spleen, which is an infection-fighting organ located just below your left rib cage;

- Red spots on the soles of your feet or the palms of your hands (Janeway **lesions**);
- Red, tender spots under the skin of your fingers or toes (Osler's nodes);
- Tiny purple or red spots, called **petechiae** on the skin, in the whites of your eyes or inside your mouth.

Causes

Endocarditis occurs when germs, usually bacteria, enter your bloodstream, travel to your heart, and attach to abnormal heart valves or damaged heart tissue. Fungi or other germs also may cause endocarditis.

Usually, your immune system destroys any harmful bacteria that enter your bloodstream. However, bacteria that live in your mouth, throat or other parts of your body, such as your skin or your gut, can sometimes cause endocarditis under the right circumstances. Bacteria, fungi and other germs that cause endocarditis might enter your bloodstream through:

- Improper dental care. Proper toothbrushing and flossing help prevent **gum** disease. If you don't take good care of your teeth and gums, brushing could cause unhealthy gums to bleed, giving bacteria a chance to enter your bloodstream. Some dental procedures that can cut your gums also may allow bacteria to enter your bloodstream.
- Catheters. Bacteria can enter your body through a thin tube that doctors sometimes use to inject or remove fluid from the body (catheter). This is more likely to occur if the catheter is in place for a long period of time. For example, you may have a catheter if you need long-term **dialysis**.
- Illegal **IV** drug use. Contaminated needles and syringes are a special concern for people who use illegal IV drugs, such as heroin or cocaine. Often, individuals who use these types of drugs don't have access to clean, unused needles or syringes.

Complications

In endocarditis, clumps made of germs and cell pieces form an abnormal mass in your heart. These clumps, called **vegetations**, can break loose and travel to your brain, lungs, abdominal organs, kidneys, or arms and legs. As a result, endocarditis can cause several complications, including:

- Heart problems, such as heart murmur, heart valve damage and heart failure;

- Stroke;
- Pockets of collected **pus** (abscesses) that develop in the heart, brain, lungs and other organs;
  - Blood clot in a lung artery (**pulmonary embolism**);
  - Kidney damage;
  - Enlarged spleen.

Diagnosis

Your doctor will consider your medical history, your signs and symptoms, and your test results when making a diagnosis of endocarditis. The diagnosis is usually based on several factors instead of a single positive test result or symptom. Tests used to confirm or rule out endocarditis include:

- Blood culture test. A blood culture test is used to identify any germs in your bloodstream. Blood culture test results help your doctor choose the most appropriate antibiotic or combination of antibiotics.
- **Complete blood count**. This blood test can tell your doctor if you have a lot of white blood cells, which can be a sign of infection. A complete blood count can also help diagnose low levels of healthy red blood cells (anemia), which can be a sign of endocarditis. Other blood tests also may be done to help your doctor determine the diagnosis.
- Echocardiogram. An echocardiogram uses sound waves to produce images of your heart while it's beating. This test shows how your heart's chambers and valves are pumping blood through your heart.
- Electrocardiogram (ECG or EKG). An ECG is used to measure the timing and duration of your heartbeats. It isn't specifically used to diagnose endocarditis, but it can show your doctor if something is affecting your heart's electrical activity. During an ECG, sensors that can detect your heart's electrical activity are attached to your chest, arms and legs.
- Chest X-ray. A chest X-ray can show your doctor the condition of your lungs and heart. It can help determine if endocarditis has caused heart swelling or if any infection has spread to your lungs.
- Computerized tomography (CT) scan or magnetic resonance imaging (MRI). You may need a CT scan or an MRI scan of your brain, chest or other parts of your body if your doctor thinks that infection has spread to these areas.

Treatment

Many people with endocarditis are successfully treated with antibiotics.

Sometimes, surgery may be needed to fix or replace damaged heart valves and clean up any remaining signs of the infection.

Medications

The type of medication you receive depends on what's causing the endocarditis. High doses of IV antibiotics are used to treat endocarditis caused by bacteria. If you receive IV antibiotics, you'll generally spend a week or more in the hospital so your doctor can determine if the treatment is working.

Once your fever and any severe signs and symptoms have gone away, you might be able to leave the hospital and continue IV antibiotics with visits to your doctor's office or at home with home care. You'll usually take antibiotics for several weeks to clear up the infection.

If endocarditis is caused by a fungal infection, your doctor will prescribe antifungal medication. Some people need lifelong antifungal pills to prevent endocarditis from returning.

Surgery

Heart valve surgery may be needed to treat persistent endocarditis infections or to replace a damaged valve. Surgery is also sometimes needed to treat endocarditis that's caused by a fungal infection.

Depending on your condition, your doctor may recommend repairing your damaged valve or replacing it with an artificial valve made of cow, pig or human heart tissue (biological tissue valve) or man-made materials (**prosthetic** mechanical valve).

(1168 words)

◇ **Vocabulary**

endocardium [endəʊˈkɑːdiəm] *n.* [解剖] 心内膜

lesion [ˈliːʒn] *n.* 损害，身体上的伤害

petechiae [pəˈtɪkɪˌi] *n.* 瘀点，出血点（petechia 的复数）

gum [gʌm] *n.* 牙龈，牙床；口香糖

dialysis [daɪˈæləsɪs] *n.* [医] [分化] 透析，渗析

IV is an abbreviation for intravenous 静脉注射

vegetation [ˌvedʒəˈteɪʃn] *n.* 疣状赘生物

pus [pʌs] *n.* 脓，脓汁

embolism [ˈembəlɪzəm] *n.* 血管阻塞，栓塞

pulmonary embolism 肺栓塞，肺血管阻塞症

complete blood count 全血细胞计数

prosthetic [prɒsˈθetɪk] *adj.* 假体的，非肤基的

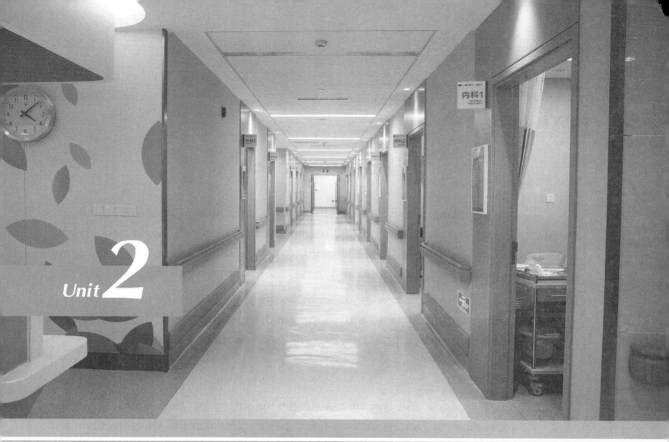

Unit **2**

Some Common Diseases of the Respiratory System

✓参考答案
✓微课等资源

Text A

Pneumonia

Pneumonia is an infection that inflames the **air sacs** in one or both lungs. The air sacs may fill with fluid or pus (**purulent** material), causing cough with **phlegm** or pus, fever, chills, and difficulty breathing. A variety of organisms, including bacteria, viruses and fungi, can cause pneumonia.

Pneumonia can range in seriousness from mild to life-threatening. It is most serious for infants and young children, people older than age 65, and people with health problems or weakened immune systems.

Symptoms

The signs and symptoms of pneumonia vary from mild to severe, depending on factors such as the type of germ causing the infection, and your age and overall health. Mild signs and symptoms often are similar to those of a cold or flu, but they last longer. Signs and symptoms of pneumonia may include:

- Chest pain when you breathe or cough;
- Confusion or changes in mental awareness (in adults age 65 and older);
- Cough, which may produce phlegm;
- Fatigue;
- Fever, sweating and shaking chills;
- Lower than normal body temperature (in adults older than age 65 and people with weak immune systems);
- Nausea, vomiting or **diarrhea**;
- Shortness of breath.

Newborns and infants may not show any sign of the infection. Or they may vomit, have a fever and cough, appear restless or tired and without energy, or have difficulty breathing and eating.

Causes

Many germs can cause pneumonia. The most common are bacteria and viruses in the air we breathe. Your body usually prevents these germs from infecting your lungs. But sometimes these germs can overpower your immune system, even if your health is generally good.

Pneumonia is classified according to the types of germs that cause it and where you got the infection.

Community-acquired pneumonia

Community-acquired pneumonia is the most common type of pneumonia. It occurs outside of hospitals or other health care facilities. It may be caused by:

• Bacteria. The most common cause of bacterial pneumonia in the U.S. is **streptococcus** pneumonia. This type of pneumonia can occur on its own or after you've had a cold or the flu. It may affect one part (lobe) of the lung, a condition called **lobar** pneumonia.

• Bacteria-like organisms. **Mycoplasma** pneumonia also can cause pneumonia. It typically produces milder symptoms than do other types of pneumonia. Walking pneumonia is an informal name given to this type of pneumonia, which typically isn't severe enough to require bed rest.

• Fungi. This type of pneumonia is most common in people with chronic health problems or weakened immune systems, and in people who have inhaled large doses of the organisms. The fungi that cause it can be found in soil or bird droppings and vary depending upon geographic location.

• Viruses, including COVID-19. Some of the viruses that cause colds and the flu can cause pneumonia. Viruses are the most common cause of pneumonia in children younger than 5 years. Viral pneumonia is usually mild. But in some cases it can become very serious. Coronavirus 2019 may cause pneumonia, which can become severe.

Hospital-acquired pneumonia

Some people catch pneumonia during a hospital stay for another illness. Hospital-acquired pneumonia can be serious because the bacteria causing it may be more resistant to antibiotics and because the people who get it are already sick. People who are on breathing machines (ventilators), often used in intensive care units, are at higher risk of this type of pneumonia.

Health care-acquired pneumonia

Health care-acquired pneumonia is a bacterial infection that occurs in people who live in long-term care facilities or who receive care in outpatient clinics, including kidney dialysis centers. Like hospital-acquired pneumonia, health care-acquired pneumonia can be caused by bacteria that are more resistant to antibiotics.

Aspiration *pneumonia*

Aspiration pneumonia occurs when you inhale food, drink, vomit or saliva into your lungs. Aspiration is more likely if something disturbs your normal **gag reflex**, such as a brain injury or swallowing problem, or excessive use of alcohol or drugs.

Diagnosis

Your doctor will start by asking about your medical history and doing a physical exam, including listening to your lungs with a **stethoscope** to check for abnormal bubbling or crackling sounds that suggest pneumonia.

If pneumonia is suspected, your doctor may recommend the following tests:

- Blood tests. Blood tests are used to confirm an infection and to try to identify the type of organism causing the infection. However, precise identification isn't always possible.
- Chest X-ray. This helps your doctor diagnose pneumonia and determine the extent and location of the infection. However, it can't tell your doctor what kind of germ is causing the pneumonia.
- Pulse **oximetry**. This measures the oxygen level in your blood. Pneumonia can prevent your lungs from moving enough oxygen into your bloodstream.
- **Sputum** test. A sample of fluid from your lungs (sputum) is taken after a deep cough and analyzed to help pinpoint the cause of the infection.

Your doctor might order additional tests if you're older than age 65, are in the hospital, or have serious symptoms or health conditions. These may include:

- CT scan. If your pneumonia isn't clearing as quickly as expected, your doctor may recommend a chest CT scan to obtain a more detailed image of your lungs.
- **Pleural** fluid culture. A fluid sample is taken by putting a needle between your ribs from the pleural area and analyzed to help determine the type of infection.

Treatment

Treatment for pneumonia involves curing the infection and preventing complications. People who have community-acquired pneumonia usually can be treated at home with medication. Although most symptoms ease in a few days or weeks, the feeling of tiredness can persist for a month or more.

Specific treatment depends on the type and severity of your pneumonia, your age and your overall health. The options include:

- Antibiotics. These medicines are used to treat bacterial pneumonia. It may take time to identify the type of bacteria causing your pneumonia and to choose the best antibiotic to treat it. If your symptoms don't improve, your doctor may recommend a different antibiotic.

- Cough medicine. This medicine may be used to calm your cough so that you can rest. Because coughing helps loosen and move fluid from your lungs, it's a good idea not to eliminate your cough completely. In addition, you should know that very few studies have looked at whether over-the-counter cough medicines lessen coughing caused by pneumonia. If you want to try a cough suppressant, use the lowest dose that helps you rest.

- Fever reducers/pain relievers. You may take these as needed for fever and discomfort. These include drugs such as aspirin, **ibuprofen** (Advil, Motrin IB,others) and **acetaminophen** (Tylenol, others).

You may need to be hospitalized if:

- You are older than age 65;
- You are confused about time, people or places;
- Your kidney function has declined;
- Your systolic blood pressure is below 90 millimeters of mercury (mm Hg) or your diastolic blood pressure is 60 mm Hg or below;
- Your breathing is rapid (30 breaths or more a minute);
- You need breathing assistance;
- Your temperature is below normal;
- Your heart rate is below 50 or above 100.

You may be admitted to the intensive care unit if you need to be placed on a breathing machine (ventilator) or if your symptoms are severe.

Children may be hospitalized if:

- They are younger than age 2 months;
- They are lethargic or excessively sleepy;
- They have trouble breathing;
- They have low blood oxygen levels;
- They appear **dehydrated.**

(1259 words)

◆ Vocabulary

air sac [eə sæk] [动] 气囊；肺泡
purulent ['pjʊərələnt] *adj.* 脓的，化脓的
phlegm [flem] *n.* 痰，黏液
diarrhea [ˌdaɪə'riːə] *n.* 腹泻(= diarrhoea)
streptococcus [ˌstreptə'kɒkəs] *n.* 链球菌
lobar ['ləʊbə(r)] *adj.* 叶的，肺叶的
mycoplasma [ˌmaɪkəʊ'plɑːzmə] *n.* [微] 支原菌，[微] 支原体
aspiration [ˌæspə'reɪʃn] *n.* [医] 吸引(术)，(体液)抽吸；渴望，抱负

gag reflex 呕反射，咽反射
stethoscope ['steθəskəʊp] *n.* 听诊器
oximetry [ɒk'sɪmɪtri] 血氧定量法，测氧法
sputum ['spjuːtəm] *n.* [生理] 痰；唾液
pleural ['plʊərəl] *adj.* 胸膜的
ibuprofen [aɪbjuː'prəʊfen] *n.* 布洛芬，异丁苯丙酸(抗炎，镇痛药)
acetaminophen [əˌsiːtə'mɪnəfen] *n.* [药] 醋氨酚，对乙酰氨基酚，退热净
dehydrate [diːhaɪ'dreɪt] *v.* 脱水；去水

◆ Exercises

Ⅰ. **Decide whether the following sentences are *True* or *False* according to the text.**

1. Bacteria, viruses and fungi can cause pneumonia.

2. The high risk groups of pneumonia include infants, young children, older people and people with weakened immune systems.

3. Mild signs and symptoms of pneumonia are similar to those of a cold or flu, but they last shorter.

4. Fatigue, fever, nausea, shortness of breath are the signs and symptoms of pneumonia.

5. Only bacteria and viruses in the air we breathe can cause pneumonia.

6. Hospital-acquired pneumonia is the most common type of pneumonia.

7. Sometimes germs can overpower your immune system, even if your body prevents them from infecting your lungs.

8. If pneumonia is suspected, blood tests, chest X-ray, etc. are recommended to confirm it.

9. People who have community-acquired pneumonia usually can be treated at hospital.

10. Serious pneumonia patients who are older than 65 or younger than 2 months, may need to be hospitalized.

II. Fill in the blanks with the proper form of words in the box.

| lobar | dehydrate | dialysis | pleural | phlegm |
| diarrhoea | nausea | stethoscope | systolic | pus |

1. _____ refers to a fluid product of inflammation.

2. _____ is the thick yellowish substance that develops in your throat and at the back of your nose when you have a cold.

3. If someone has _____ , a lot of liquid faeces comes out of their body because they are ill.

4. A checkup revealed a small tumour on the left _____ of his lung, but it had not yet metastasized.

5. _____ is a medical instrument for listening to the sounds generated inside the body.

6. People can very quickly _____ in the desert, so take plenty of water for a desert adventure.

7. _____ blood pressure refers to the peak pressure in the arteries around the time that the heart muscle contracts.

8. _____ refers to the thin serous membrane around the lungs and inner walls of the chest.

9. _____ is the condition of feeling sick and the feeling that you are going to vomit.

10. Once kidneys fail, _____ is necessary.

III. Translation: translate the passage into Chinese.

There are many components to the respiratory system. They include nose, mouth, throat (pharynx), voice box (larynx), windpipe (trachea), large airways (bronchi), small airways (bronchioles), lungs, and diaphragm.

As we breathe, oxygen enters the nose or mouth and passes the sinuses, which are hollow spaces in the skull that help regulate the temperature and humidity of the air we breathe.

From the sinuses, air passes through the trachea, also called the windpipe, and into the bronchial tubes, which are the two tubes that carry air into each lung (each one is called a bronchus). The bronchial tubes are lined with tiny hairs called cilia that move back and forth, carrying mucus up and out. Mucus is a sticky fluid that collects dust, germs and other matter that has invaded the lungs and is what we expel when we sneeze and cough.

The bronchial tubes split up again to carry air into the lobes of each lung. The right lung has three lobes while the left lung has only two, to accommodate room for the heart. The lobes are filled with small, spongy sacs called alveoli, which is where the exchange of oxygen and carbon dioxide occurs.

The alveolar walls are extremely thin (about 0.2 micrometers) and are composed of a single layer of tissues called epithelial cells and tiny blood vessels called pulmonary capillaries. Blood in the capillaries picks up oxygen and drops off carbon dioxide. The oxygenated blood then makes its way to the pulmonary veins. These veins carry oxygen-rich blood to the left side of the heart, where it is pumped to all parts of the body. The carbon dioxide the blood left behind moves into the alveoli and gets expelled in our exhaled breath.

The diaphragm, a dome-shaped muscle at the bottom of the lungs, controls breathing and separates the chest cavity from the abdominal cavity. When air gets taken in, the diaphragm tightens and moves downward, making more space for the lungs to fill with air and expand. During exhalation, the diaphragm expands and compresses the lungs, forcing air out.

(358 words)

IV. Give a presentation.

Dictate the causes, symptoms, treatments, etc. of Pneumonia in English with 3—4 students. Try to use the formal expression, especially related medical terminology when you make your presentation.

V. Write a job application.

请根据下列内容,给某网站的 Richard 女士写一封求职信。

某网站暑假期间招聘一名会两门外语的社区卫生助理实习生,你应聘的理由:懂西班牙语和英语,对卫生保健很感兴趣;大一在当地的社区医院做过助理护理师;去年夏天,为 Louis 医生做过医疗记录助手,整理和管理病人信息。

Text B

Non-Small Cell Lung Cancer

Lung cancer is cancer that forms in tissues of the lung, usually in the cells that line the **air passages**. It is the leading cause of cancer death in both men and women. There are two main types: small cell lung cancer (SCLC) and **non-small cell lung cancer** (NSCLC). These two types grow differently and are treated differently. Non-small cell lung cancer is the more common type.

Most people who have lung cancer have NSCLC. Although it's serious, treatment can sometimes stop it from getting worse. There are things you can do to help you feel better, too. People who smoke or who breathe a lot of smoke are most likely to get NSCLC. Many of them are over 65.

There are four kinds of NSCLC tumors:

• **Adenocarcinoma** starts in cells in your air sacs that make **mucus** and other substances, often in the outer parts of your lungs. It's the most common kind of lung cancer among both smokers and nonsmokers and people under 45. It often grows more slowly than other lung cancers.

• **Squamous cell carcinoma** starts in cells that line the inner airways of the lungs. About a quarter of lung cancers are this kind.

• Large cell (undifferentiated) carcinoma grows and spreads more quickly. That can make it tougher to treat. It's about 10% of lung cancers.

• **Adenosquamous carcinoma** is relatively rare and generally develops in the outer part of the lungs. Smoking can increase the risk of its development.

The treatments your doctor suggests will depend on how far your lung cancer has spread.

Causes

Doctors aren't sure exactly what causes this disease. Many people who get it have smoked or been around smoke. Other things that make lung cancer more likely are:

• **Radon**, a radioactive gas found naturally in soil and rocks;
• **Asbestos**;
• Mineral and metal dust;
• Chronic obstructive pulmonary disease (COPD);

- Pulmonary **fibrosis**;
- Air pollution;
- Radiation treatment to your chest or breast;
- HIV/AIDS.

Symptoms

You may not notice symptoms in the early stages. Like other types of lung cancer, symptoms can include:

- Coughing that lasts or gets worse;
- Chest pain that often hurts more when you cough, laugh, or take deep breaths;
- **Hoarseness** or voice changes;
- Harsh, **raspy** sounds when you breathe;
- Wheezing;
- Weight loss, little appetite;
- Coughing up blood or mucus;
- Shortness of breath;
- Feeling weak or tired;
- Lasting lung problems, like **bronchitis** or pneumonia.

If the cancer spreads to other parts of the body, you may have:

- Bone pain;
- Headache;
- Dizziness or balance problems;
- Numbness or weakness in an arm or a leg;
- Yellow skin or eyes.

Diagnosis

First, your doctor will talk with you and ask questions like:

- When did you first notice problems?
- How have you been feeling?
- Are you coughing or wheezing?
- Does anything make your symptoms better or worse?
- What do you do for a living?
- Do you, or did you, smoke?
- Has anyone in your family had lung cancer?

They'll also give you a physical exam. You will need tests, too.

Imaging tests help your doctor find tumors inside your lungs. They can also show whether the cancer has spread.

- X-rays use low doses of radiation to make images of structures inside your body.
- MRI, or magnetic resonance imaging, shows blood flow, organs, and structures.
- Ultrasound creates a picture by bouncing sound waves off tissues inside you.
- **PET** scans use a radioactive compound or tracer that collects where your cells are very active.
- CT scans are powerful X-rays that make detailed pictures of the tissue and the blood vessels in the lung.

Sputum cytology is a lab test that checks the mucus you cough up for cancer cells.

Fine-needle aspiration biopsy takes cells from an abnormal growth or the fluid in your lungs. Your doctor may want to look inside your lungs and chest using a thin, flexible tube with a light and tiny camera. They can do this a few different ways:

- **Bronchoscopy** goes through your nose or mouth and into your lungs.
- **Endobronchial** ultrasound uses bronchoscopy with an ultrasound placed at the tip of the tube to look at lymph nodes and other structures.
- **Endoscopic** ultrasound is like the endobronchial ultrasound, but your doctor puts the endoscope down your throat into the esophagus.
- **Thoracoscopy** uses a few small cuts along your side to look at the outside of your lung and the tissue around it.
- **Mediastinoscopy** makes a small cut just above your breastbone, in the space between your lungs.

Based on what your doctor finds, they'll assign a stage, describing where the cancer is. That will help your medical team figure out the best treatment for you. You'll want to know what each stage means:

- Occult stage: "**Occult**" means "hidden". Cancer cells are in lung fluid or sputum, but the doctor can't find where the cancer is in your lungs.
- Stage 0: Cancer cells are in the lining of your airways.
- Stage Ⅰ: A small tumor is in only one lung. The cancer hasn't spread to lymph nodes.
- Stage Ⅱ: A larger tumor is in one lung, or the cancer has spread to nearby lymph nodes.

• Stage Ⅲ: Cancer in one lung has spread to farther lymph nodes or into nearby structures.

• Stage Ⅳ: Cancer has spread to both lungs, to fluid around the lungs, or to other parts of the body, such as the brain and liver.

Treatment

Doctors treat this kind of lung cancer in two ways: They target the cancer itself, and they try to make you feel better. Your doctor may suggest a combination of treatments, depending on what kind of cancer you have and where it is.

Surgery. If you're in an early stage, your doctor will probably recommend surgery to take out the cancer. You could have a part or all of your lung removed. Other types of surgery destroy cancer cells by freezing them or using a heated probe or needle.

Radiation. It can kill cancer cells that remain after surgery. The radiation comes either from a high-energy beam aimed at the cancer from outside of your body using a special machine, or from a radioactive substance put inside your body in or near the cancer.

Chemotherapy. Whether you get it as pills or with a needle in a vein or muscle, the drugs travel throughout your body to kill the cancer. Your doctor might put it in your spinal fluid, a specific organ, or a space inside your body to target cancer cells in that area.

Targeted therapy. These drugs and antibodies stop cancer cells from growing and spreading in very specific ways. Because of how they work, they usually harm normal cells less than radiation and chemo.

Laser and photodynamic therapy (PDT). This technique uses a special laser light to "turn on" special drugs that cancer cells have absorbed. This kills them and helps avoid damage to healthy tissue.

Clinical trials. Scientists are studying new ways to treat cancer. Check the National Cancer Institute's website and ask your doctor if a clinical trial would be a good fit for you, what you should consider, and how to sign up.

（1231 words）

Vocabulary

air passage 气道

non-small cell lung cancer 非小细胞型肺癌

adenocarcinoma [ˌædɪnəʊˌkɑːsɪˈnəʊmə] n. [肿瘤] 腺癌

mucus [ˈmjuːkəs] n. 黏液

carcinoma [ˌkɑːsɪˈnəʊmə] n. [肿瘤] 癌

squamous cell carcinoma 鳞状细胞癌

adenosquamous carcinoma 腺鳞癌

radon [ˈreɪdɒn] n. [化学] 氡

asbestos [æsˈbestɒs] n. 石棉 adj. 石棉的

fibrosis [faɪˈbrəʊsɪs] n. [医] 纤维化，[病理] 纤维变性

hoarse [hɔːs] adj. 嘶哑的

raspy [ˈrɑːspi] adj. 刺耳的，易怒的；粗糙的

bronchitis [brɒŋˈkaɪtɪs] n. [内科] 支气管炎

PET（positron emission tomography）正电子发射扫描

cytology [saɪˈtɒlədʒi] n. 细胞学

bronchoscopy [bˈrɒntʃəskəpi] n. [耳鼻喉] 支气管镜检查

endobronchial [endəʊbˈrɒnkɪəl] adj. 支气管内的

endoscopic [ˌendəsˈkɒpɪk] adj. 内窥镜的，用内窥镜检查的

thoracoscopy [θɔːrəˈkɒskəpi] n. 胸腔镜检查，胸腔镜

mediastinoscopy [mediəsˈtɪnɒskəpi] n. [临床] 纵隔镜检查

occult [əˈkʌlt] adj. 神秘的，(疾病)不伴随可见迹象(或症状)的

chemotherapy [ˌkiːməʊˈθerəpi] n. [临床] 化学疗法

Exercises

Ⅰ. **Decide whether the following sentences are *True* or *False* according to the text.**

1. People who smoke or who breathe a lot of smoke are most likely to get SCLC. Many of them are over 65.

2. Causes of NSCLC include radioactive gas, pulmonary fibrosis and radiation, but HIV/AIDS is excluded.

3. Symptoms of NSCLC include coughing, chest pain, hoarseness, wheezing, and coughing up blood or mucus, etc.

4. Sputum cytology is a lab test that checks the mucus you cough up for cancer cells.

5. If a small tumor is in only one lung and has spread to lymph nodes, this is in Stage Ⅰ.

6. Targeted therapy only harms cancer cells instead of normal cells.

7. The radiation comes either from a high-energy beam from outside of your body, or from a radioactive substance put inside your body in or near the cancer.

8. If cancer in one lung has spread to other parts of the body, such as the brain and

liver, it is in Stage Ⅲ.

9. Yellow skin and harsh, raspy sounds when you breathe are not typical symptoms of NSCLC.

10. Adenosquamous carcinoma is relatively rare and generally develops in the inner part of the lungs.

Ⅱ. **Fill in the blanks with the proper form of words in the box.**

sputum	endoscopy	pulmonary	cytology	adenocarcinoma	bronchoscopy
mediastinoscopy		chemotherapy		aspiration	carcinoma

1. _____ is the one cell type of primary lung tumor that occurs more often in non-smokers and in smokers who have quit.

2. Basal cell _____ occurs most often on areas of the skin that are exposed to the sun, such as your head and neck.

3. _____ embolism is a blockage in one of the pulmonary arteries in your lungs, which in most cases is caused by blood clots that travel to the lungs from deep veins in the legs.

4. A non-productive cough does not expel _____ from the respiratory tract.

5. _____ is the study of the structure of all normal and abnormal components of cells and the changes, movements, and transformations of such components.

6. Often, fine-needle _____ is done using ultrasound to guide accurate placement of the needle.

7. _____ is a method of direct examination of the trachea and bronchi by means of a special instrument.

8. An _____ is a procedure used in medicine to look inside the body.

9. The accuracy rate of _____ is 93.33% for diagnosing enlarged lymph nodes.

10. _____ refers to the treatment of disease with chemicals or drugs.

Ⅲ. **Translation: translate the passage into Chinese.**

Advanced lung cancer means that the cancer has spread from where it started in the lung. It is also called metastatic cancer. The cancer might also cause fluid that contains cancer cells to collect around the lung. This is called fluid on the lung or a pleural effusion.

Unfortunately advanced cancer can't usually be cured. But treatment might control it, help symptoms, and improve your quality of life for a while. A cancer might be advanced when it is first diagnosed. Or it may come back some time after you were first treated. This is called recurrent cancer.

Locally advanced cancer is cancer that has spread into tissues around the lungs. For example, it may grow into an airway, the chest wall or the membranes that surround the lung (the pleura). A cancer that has spread to another part of the body is called a secondary cancer or metastasis. Not all lung cancers will spread. But if the cancer does spread, there are certain parts of the body that it is more likely to go to. The most common areas for lung cancer to spread to are nearby lymph nodes, the brain, bones, the liver, the adrenal glands (small hormone glands just above your kidney), other parts of the lung or the other lung.

Finding out that you can't be cured is distressing and can be a shock. It's common to feel uncertain and anxious. It's normal to not be able to think about anything else. Many people want to know what the outlook is and how their cancer will develop. This is different for each person. Your cancer specialist has all the information about you and your cancer. They're the best person to discuss this with.

(293 words)

IV. Give a presentation.

Dictate the causes, symptoms, treatments, etc. of Non-Small Cell Lung Cancer in English with 3—4 students. Try to use the formal expression, especially related medical terminology when you make your presentation.

V. Write an appreciation letter.

请根据下列内容写一封见习感谢信。

在实习结束时,请给 Richard 女士写一封见习感谢信,感谢她给你实习的机会,同时概述一下自己在实习中的所思所想。

Text C

Asthma

Asthma is a condition in which your airways narrow and swell and may produce extra mucus. This can make breathing difficult and trigger coughing, a whistling sound (**wheezing**) when you breathe out and shortness of breath. For some people, asthma is a minor nuisance. For others, it can be a major problem that interferes with daily activities and may lead to a life-threatening asthma attack. Asthma can't be cured, but its symptoms can be controlled. Because asthma often changes over time, it's important that you work with your doctor to track your signs and symptoms and adjust your treatment as needed.

Symptoms

Asthma symptoms vary from person to person. You may have infrequent asthma attacks, have symptoms only at certain times—such as when exercising—or have symptoms all the time. Asthma signs and symptoms include:

- Shortness of breath;
- Chest tightness or pain;
- Wheezing when exhaling, which is a common sign of asthma in children;
- Trouble sleeping caused by shortness of breath, coughing or wheezing;
- Coughing or wheezing attacks that are worsened by a respiratory virus, such as a cold or the flu.

Signs that your asthma is probably worsening include:

- Asthma signs and symptoms that are more frequent and bothersome;
- Increasing difficulty breathing, as measured with a device used to check how well your lungs are working (**peak flow meter**);
- The need to use a quick-relief **inhaler** more often.

For some people, asthma signs and symptoms flare up in certain situations:

- Exercise-induced asthma, which may be worse when the air is cold and dry;

- Occupational asthma, triggered by workplace **irritants** such as chemical fumes, gases or dust;
- Allergy-induced asthma, triggered by airborne substances, such as **pollen, mold spores, cockroach** waste, or particles of skin and dried saliva shed by pets (pet dander).

Causes

It isn't clear why some people get asthma and others don't, but it's probably due to a combination of environmental and inherited (genetic) factors.

Exposure to various irritants and substances that trigger allergies (allergens) can trigger signs and symptoms of asthma. Asthma triggers are different from person to person and can include:

- Airborne **allergens**, such as pollen, **dust mites**, mold spores, pet **dander** or particles of cockroach waste;
- Respiratory infections, such as the common cold;
- Physical activity;
- Cold air;
- Air pollutants and irritants, such as smoke;
- Certain medications, including **beta blockers**, aspirin, and **nonsteroidal** anti-inflammatory drugs;
- Strong emotions and stress;
- **Sulfites** and **preservatives** added to some types of foods and beverages, including shrimp, dried fruit, processed potatoes, beer and wine;
- **Gastroesophageal reflux** disease (GERD), a condition in which stomach acids back up into your throat.

Diagnosis

Physical exam
Your doctor will perform a physical exam to rule out other possible conditions, such as a respiratory infection or chronic obstructive pulmonary disease (COPD). Your doctor will also ask you questions about your signs and symptoms and about any other health problems.

Tests to measure lung function
You may be given lung function tests to determine how much air moves in and out as you breathe. These tests may include:

- **Spirometry**. This test estimates the narrowing of your **bronchial tubes** by checking how much air you can exhale after a deep breath and how fast you can breathe out.

• Peak flow. A peak flow meter is a simple device that measures how hard you can breathe out. Lower than usual peak flow readings are a sign that your lungs may not be working as well and that your asthma may be getting worse.

Additional tests

Other tests to diagnose asthma include:

• **Methacholine** challenge. Methacholine is a known asthma trigger. When inhaled, it will cause your airways to narrow slightly. If you react to the methacholine, you likely have asthma. This test may be used even if your initial lung function test is normal.

• Imaging tests. A chest X-ray can help identify any structural abnormalities or diseases (such as infection) that can cause or aggravate breathing problems.

• Allergy testing. Allergy tests can be performed by a skin test or blood test. They tell you if you're allergic to pets, dust, mold or pollen. If allergy triggers are identified, your doctor may recommend allergy shots.

• **Nitric oxide** test. This test measures the amount of the gas nitric oxide in your breath. When your airways are inflamed—a sign of asthma—you may have higher than normal nitric oxide levels. This test isn't widely available.

• Sputum **eosinophils**. This test looks for certain white blood cells (eosinophils) in the mixture of saliva and mucus (sputum) you **discharge** during coughing. Eosinophils are present when symptoms develop and become visible when stained with a rose-colored dye.

• Provocative testing for exercise and cold-induced asthma. In these tests, your doctor measures your airway obstruction before and after you perform vigorous physical activity or take several breaths of cold air.

How asthma is classified

To classify your asthma severity, your doctor will consider how often you have signs and symptoms and how severe they are. Your doctor will also consider the results of your physical exam and diagnostic tests. Asthma is classified into four general categories:

• Mild intermittent: Mild symptoms up to two days a week and up to two nights a month;

• Mild persistent: Symptoms more than twice a week, but no more than once in a single day;

- Moderate persistent: Symptoms once a day and more than one night a week;
- Severe persistent: Symptoms throughout the day on most days and frequently at night.

Treatment

Prevention and long-term control are key to stopping asthma attacks before they start. Treatment usually involves learning to recognize your triggers, taking steps to avoid triggers and tracking your breathing to make sure your medications are keeping symptoms under control. In case of an asthma flare-up, you may need to use a quick-relief inhaler.

Medications

The right medications for you depend on a number of things—your age, symptoms, asthma triggers and what works best to keep your asthma under control. Preventive, long-term control medications reduce the swelling (inflammation) in your airways that leads to symptoms. Quick-relief inhalers (bronchodilators) quickly open swollen airways that are limiting breathing. In some cases, allergy medications are necessary.

Long-term asthma control medications, generally taken daily, are the cornerstone of asthma treatment. These medications keep asthma under control on a day-to-day basis and make it less likely you'll have an asthma attack. Quick-relief (rescue) medications are used as needed for rapid, short-term symptom relief during an asthma attack. They may also be used before exercise if your doctor recommends it. If you have an asthma flare-up, a quick-relief inhaler can ease your symptoms right away. But you shouldn't need to use your quick-relief inhaler very often if your long-term control medications are working properly.

Bronchial thermoplasty

This treatment is used for severe asthma that doesn't improve with inhaled **corticosteroids** or other long-term asthma medications. It isn't widely available nor right for everyone.

During bronchial thermoplasty, your doctor heats the insides of the airways in the lungs with an electrode. The heat reduces the smooth muscle inside the airways. This limits the ability of the airways to tighten, making breathing easier and possibly reducing asthma attacks. The therapy is generally done over three outpatient visits.

(1228 words)

◆ **Vocabulary**

asthma ['æsmə] *n.* [内科][中医] 哮喘, 气喘

wheeze [wiːz] *v.* 喘息, 喘息地说

peak flow meter 最大流量计

inhaler [ɪn'heɪlə(r)] *n.* [临床] 吸入器, 空气过滤器

irritant ['ɪrɪtənt] *n.* [医] 刺激物, 刺激剂

pollen ['pɒlən] *n.* 花粉

mold spore 霉菌孢子

cockroach ['kɒkrəutʃ] *n.* 蟑螂

allergen ['ælədʒən] *n.* [医] 过敏原

mite [maɪt] *n.* 小虫, 螨; 微粒, 微小的东西

dust mite 尘螨

dander ['dændə(r)] *n.* 头皮屑, 羽毛屑
　　v. 漫步, 闲逛

beta blockers β-受体阻滞药

steroidal [stə'rɔɪdəl] *adj.* 甾族的, 甾体的

sulfite ['sʌlfaɪt] *n.* [无化] 亚硫酸盐 (= sulphite)

preservative [prɪ'zɜːrvətɪv] *n.* 防腐的, [助剂] 防腐剂, 保存剂

gastroesophageal ['gæstrəuɪˌsɒfə'dʒiːəl] *adj.* 胃食管的

reflux ['riːflʌks] *n.* 逆流, 退潮

spirometry [spaɪə'rɒmɪtri] *n.* 呼吸量测定法, 肺(活)量测定法

bronchial ['brɒŋkiəl] *adj.* 支气管的

bronchial tubes 支气管小支气管

methacholine [meθeɪ'kəulɪn] *n.* 乙酰甲胆碱, 醋甲胆碱

nitric oxide ['naɪtrɪk 'ɒksaɪd] *n.* 一氧化氮

eosinophil [ˌiːəʊ'sɪnəfɪl] *adj.* 嗜酸性的
　　n. 嗜酸性粒细胞

discharge [dɪs'tʃɑːdʒ] *n.* (液体等) 排出, 排出物　*v.* 释放, 排出

corticosteroid [ˌkɔːtɪkəʊ'stɪərɔɪd] *n.* [生化] 皮质类固醇, 皮质甾(类)

Text D

Bronchitis

Bronchitis is an inflammation of the lining of your bronchial tubes, which carry air to and from your lungs. People who have bronchitis often cough up thickened mucus, which can be discolored. Bronchitis may be either acute or chronic. Often developing from a cold or other respiratory infection, acute bronchitis is very common. Chronic bronchitis, a more serious condition, is a constant irritation or inflammation of the lining of the bronchial tubes, often due to smoking. Acute bronchitis, also called a chest cold, usually improves within a week to 10 days without lasting effects, although the cough may linger for weeks. However, if you have repeated **bouts** of bronchitis, you may have chronic bronchitis, which requires medical attention. Chronic bronchitis is one of the conditions included in chronic obstructive pulmonary disease (COPD).

Symptoms

For either acute bronchitis or chronic bronchitis, signs and symptoms may include:

- Cough;
- Production of mucus (sputum), which can be clear, white, yellowish-gray or green in color—rarely, it may be **streaked** with blood;
- Fatigue;
- Shortness of breath;
- Slight fever and chills;
- Chest discomfort.

If you have acute bronchitis, you might have cold symptoms, such as a mild headache or body aches. If you have chronic bronchitis, you're likely to have periods when your cough or other symptoms worsen.

Causes

Acute bronchitis is usually caused by viruses, typically the same viruses that cause colds and flu (influenza). Antibiotics don't kill viruses, so this type of medication isn't useful in most cases of bronchitis.

The most common cause of chronic bronchitis is cigarette smoking. Air pollution and dust or toxic gases in the environment or workplace can also contribute to the condition.

Risk factors

Factors that increase your risk of bronchitis include:

• Cigarette smoke. People who smoke or who live with a smoker are at higher risk of both acute bronchitis and chronic bronchitis.

• Low resistance. This may result from another acute illness, such as a cold, or from a chronic condition that compromises your immune system. Older adults, infants and young children have greater vulnerability to infection.

• Exposure to irritants on the job. Your risk of developing bronchitis is greater if you work around certain lung irritants, such as grains or textiles, or are exposed to chemical fumes.

• **Gastric** reflux. Repeated bouts of severe heartburn can irritate your throat and make you more prone to developing bronchitis.

Complications

Although a single episode of bronchitis usually isn't cause for concern, it can lead to pneumonia in some people. Repeated bouts of bronchitis, however, may mean that you have chronic obstructive pulmonary disease (COPD).

Prevention

To reduce your risk of bronchitis, follow these tips:

• Avoid cigarette smoke. Cigarette smoke increases your risk of chronic bronchitis.

• Get vaccinated. Many cases of acute bronchitis result from influenza, a virus. Getting a yearly flu vaccine can help protect you from getting the flu. You may also want to consider vaccination that protects against some types of pneumonia.

• Wash your hands. To reduce your risk of catching a viral infection, wash your hands frequently and get in the habit of using alcohol-based hand **sanitizers**.

• Wear a surgical mask. If you have COPD, you might consider wearing a face mask at work if you're exposed to dust or fumes, and when you're going to be among crowds, such as while traveling.

Diagnosis

During the first few days of illness, it can be difficult to distinguish the signs and symptoms of bronchitis from those of a common cold. During the physical exam, your doctor will use a stethoscope to listen closely to your lungs as you breathe. In some cases, your doctor may suggest the following tests:

• Chest X-ray. A chest X-ray can help determine if you have pneumonia or another condition that may explain your cough. This is especially important if you ever were or currently are a smoker.

• Sputum tests. Sputum is the mucus that you cough up from your lungs. It can be tested to see if you have illnesses that could be helped by antibiotics. Sputum can also be tested for signs of allergies.

• Pulmonary function test. During a pulmonary function test, you blow into a device called a **spirometer**, which measures how much air your lungs can hold and how quickly you can get air out of your lungs. This test checks for signs of asthma or **emphysema**.

Treatment

Most cases of acute bronchitis get better without treatment, usually within a couple of weeks.

Medications

Because most cases of bronchitis are caused by viral infections, antibiotics aren't effective. However, if your doctor suspects that you have a bacterial infection, he or she may prescribe an antibiotic. In some circumstances, your doctor may recommend other medications, including:

• Cough medicine. If your cough keeps you from sleeping, you might try cough suppressants at bedtime.

• Other medications. If you have allergies, asthma or chronic obstructive pulmonary disease (COPD), your doctor may recommend an **inhaler** and other medications to reduce inflammation and open narrowed passages in your lungs.

Therapies

If you have chronic bronchitis, you may benefit from pulmonary rehabilitation—a breathing exercise program in which a respiratory therapist teaches you how to breathe more easily and increase your ability to exercise.

Lifestyle and home remedies

To help you feel better, you may want to try the following self-care measures:

• Avoid lung irritants. Don't smoke. Wear a mask when the air is polluted or if you're exposed to irritants, such as paint or household cleaners with strong fumes.

• Use a **humidifier**. Warm, moist air helps relieve coughs and loosens mucus in your airways. But be sure to clean the humidifier according to the manufacturer's recommendations to avoid the growth of bacteria and fungi in the water container.

• Consider a face mask outside. If cold air aggravates your cough and causes shortness of breath, put on a cold-air face mask before you go outside.

(992 words)

◇ **Vocabulary**

bouts [baʊts] *n.* 发作；来回一次（bout 的复数）

streak [striːk] *vi.* 加上条纹；飞跑，疾驶

gastric ['gæstrɪk] *adj.* 胃的，胃部的

sanitizer ['sænɪtaɪzə(r)] *n.* 消毒杀菌剂（= sanitiser）

spirometer [spaɪ'rɒmɪtə(r)] *n.* 呼吸量计，[生理] 肺活量计

emphysema [ˌemfɪ'siːmə] *n.* [临床] 气肿，肺气肿

humidifier [hjuː'mɪdɪfaɪə(r)] *n.* 增湿器，加湿器

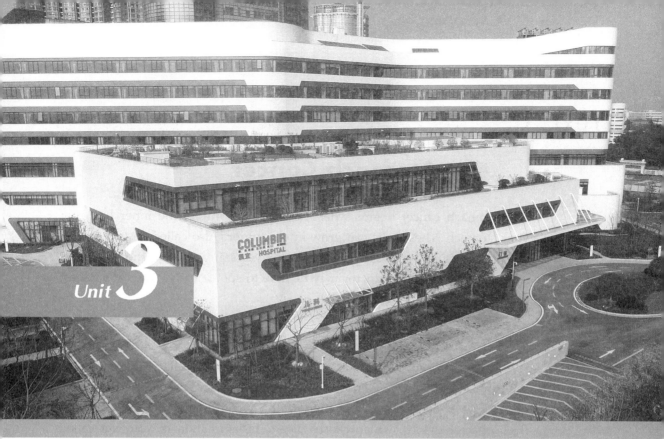

Unit **3**

Some Common Diseases of the Digestive System

✓参考答案
✓微课等资源

Text A

Stomach Cancer

Stomach cancer begins when cancer cells form in the inner lining of your stomach. These cells can grow into a tumor. Also called gastric cancer, the disease usually grows slowly over many years. If you know the symptoms it causes, you and your doctor may be able to spot it early, when it's easiest to treat.

Causes

Scientists don't know exactly what makes cancer cells start growing in the stomach. But they do know a few things that can raise your risk for the disease. One of them is infection with a common bacteria, H. **pylori** (Helicobacter pylori), which causes ulcers. Inflammation in your **gut** called **gastritis**, a certain type of long-lasting anemia called **pernicious anemia**, and growths in your stomach called **polyps** also can make you more likely to get cancer. Other things that seem to play a role in raising the risk include:

- Smoking;
- Being overweight or obese;
- A diet high in smoked, **pickled**, or salty foods;
- Stomach surgery for an ulcer;
- Type-A blood;
- Epstein-Barr virus infection;
- Certain genes;
- Working in coal, metal, timber, or rubber industries;
- Exposure to asbestos.

Symptoms

Early on, stomach cancer may cause:

- Indigestion;
- Feeling bloated after you eat a meal;
- Heartburn;
- Slight nausea;
- Loss of appetite.

Just having indigestion or heartburn after a meal doesn't mean you have cancer. But if you feel these symptoms a lot, talk to your doctor. They can see if you have other risk factors and test you to look for any problems.

As stomach tumors grow, you may have more serious symptoms, such as:

- Stomach pain;
- Blood in your stool;
- Vomiting;
- Weight loss for no reason;
- Trouble swallowing;
- Yellowish eyes or skin;
- Swelling in your stomach;
- **Constipation** or diarrhea;
- Weakness or feeling tired;
- Heartburn.

Diagnosis

If you're at higher risk for it, talk to your doctor to see how to keep an eye out for it. To find out if you have stomach cancer, your doctor starts with a physical exam. They'll also ask about your medical history to see if you have any risk factors for stomach cancer or any family members who've had it. Then, they might give you some tests, including:

- Blood tests to look for signs of cancer in your body.
- Upper endoscopy. Your doctor will put a thin, flexible tube with a small camera down your throat to look into your stomach.
- Upper **GI** series test. You'll drink a chalky liquid with a substance called barium. The fluid coats your stomach and makes it show up more clearly on X-rays.
- CT scan. This is a powerful X-ray that makes detailed pictures of the inside of your body.
- Biopsy. Your doctor takes a small piece of tissue from your stomach to look at under a microscope for signs of cancer cells. They might do this during an endoscopy.

Treatment

Treatment can fight stomach cancer. The treatment you and your doctor choose will depend on how long you've had the disease or how much it has spread in your body, called the stage of your cancer:

Stage 0. This is when the inside lining of your stomach has a group of unhealthy cells that may turn into cancer. Surgery usually cures it. Your doctor may remove part or all of your stomach, as well as nearby lymph nodes—small organs that are part of your body's germ-fighting system.

Stage Ⅰ. At this point, you have a tumor in your stomach's lining, and it may have spread into your lymph nodes. As with Stage 0, you'll likely have surgery to remove part or all of your stomach and nearby lymph nodes. You might also get chemotherapy or chemoradiation. Chemotherapy uses drugs to attack cancer cells. Chemoradiation is chemo plus radiation therapy, which destroys cancer cells with beams of high energy.

Stage Ⅱ. Cancer has spread into deeper layers of the stomach and maybe into nearby lymph nodes. Surgery to remove part or all of your stomach, as well as nearby lymph nodes, is still the main treatment. You're very likely to get chemo or chemoradiation beforehand, and you might get one of them after, too.

Stage Ⅲ. The cancer may now be in all layers of the stomach, as well as other organs close by, like the spleen or **colon**. Or, it may be smaller but reach deep into your lymph nodes. You usually have surgery to remove your entire stomach, along with chemo or chemoradiation. This can sometimes cure it. If not, it can at least help with symptoms. If you're too sick for surgery, you may get chemo, radiation, or both, depending on what your body can handle.

Stage Ⅳ. In this last stage, cancer has spread far and wide to organs like the liver, lungs, or brain. It's much harder to cure, but your doctor can help manage it and give you some relief from symptoms.

If the tumor blocks part of your GI system, you may get:

• A procedure that destroys part of the tumor with a laser on an endoscope, a thin tube that slides down your throat.

• A thin metal tube called a stent that can keep things flowing. You can get one of these between your stomach and esophagus or between your stomach and small intestine.

• Gastric bypass surgery to create a route around the tumor.

• Surgery to remove part of your stomach.

Chemo, radiation, or both may be used at this stage, too. You might also get targeted therapy. These drugs attack cancer cells, but leave healthy ones alone, which may mean fewer side effects.

Prevention

Treat stomach infections. If you have ulcers from an H. pylori infection, get treatment. Antibiotics can kill the bacteria, and other drugs will heal the sores in the lining of your stomach to cut your risk of cancer.

Eat healthy. Get more fresh fruits and vegetables on your plate every day. They're high in fiber and in some vitamins that can lower your cancer risk. Avoid very salty, pickled, cured, or smoked foods like hot dogs, processed lunch meats, or smoked cheeses.

Don't smoke. Your stomach cancer risk doubles if you use tobacco.

Watch aspirin or NSAID use. If you take daily aspirin to prevent heart problems or NSAID drugs for **arthritis**, talk to your doctor about how these drugs might affect your stomach. Though stomach cancer is the fourth most common cancer in the world, the number of cases has dropped over the past several decades.

Check on ulcers. Helicobacter pylori (H. pylori) is a common bacteria. It doesn't always make people sick, but it can infect your stomach lining and cause ulcers.

Make a move. Exercise is an everyday habit that pays off from head to toe. Being fit and active can lower your risk for many different types of cancers and other health problems.

Check on your weight. People who are overweight may be more likely to get stomach cancer.

Consider genetic testing. Does stomach cancer run in your family? A genetic test can tell you if you carry certain genes that make you more sensitive to stomach cancer, including the **CDH1 gene** and **Lynch syndrome**.

（1228 words）

◆ **Vocabulary**

pylori ［paɪˈlɒraɪ］ n. 幽门（pylorus 的复数）
gut ［gʌt］ n. 内脏；肠子
gastritis ［gæˈstraɪtɪs］ n. ［内科］胃炎
pernicious ［pəˈnɪʃəs］ adj. 有害的，恶性的；

致命的，险恶的
pernicious anemia ［内科］恶性贫血
polyp ［ˈpɒlɪp］ n. 息肉；珊瑚虫，水螅虫
pickle ［ˈpɪkl］ n. 泡菜，盐卤，腌制食品

constipation [ˌkɒnstɪ'peɪʃn] *n.* [临床] 便秘；受限制

GI is the short form of gastrointestinal. *adj.* 胃肠的

colon ['kəʊlən] *n.* [解剖] 结肠；冒号

arthritis [ɑː'θraɪtɪs] *n.* [外科] 关节炎

CDH1 gene 上皮-钙粘连素基因

Lynch syndrome 林奇综合征

Exercises

Ⅰ. **Decide whether the following sentences are *True* or *False* according to the text.**

1. Scientists already know exactly what makes gastric cancer, that's why they can treat it.

2. Causes of stomach cancer include H. pylori, overweight, certain genes, etc. However, salty foods is not a risk factor.

3. Indigestion, heartburn, constipation, blood in your stool are some symptoms of gastric cancer.

4. Barium can coat your stomach and makes it show up more clearly on X-rays.

5. If cancer has spread into deeper layers of the stomach and maybe into nearby lymph nodes, it is in Stage Ⅰ.

6. Even if your stomach cancer is in Stage Ⅳ, your doctor can easily cure it.

7. If you have ulcers caused by H. pylori infection, you should take some antibiotics to treat it to prevent stomach cancer.

8. Epstein-Barr virus infection is likely to cause stomach cancer, so do smoking and certain genes.

9. People who are overweight or obese may be more unlikely to get stomach cancer.

10. Pickled and smoked foods are risk factors to stomach cancer, but exposure to asbestos is excluded.

Ⅱ. **Fill in the blanks with the proper form of words in the box.**

polyp	colon	gastric	gut	anemia
pylori	constipation	gastrointestinal	gastritis	arthritis

1. _____ ulcer is an ulcer of the mucous membrane of the stomach.

2. The majority of ulcers are caused by infection with Helicobacter _____ bacteria.

3. Toxins can leak from the _____ into the bloodstream.

4. _____ is an inflammation disease of the mucosa of the stomach.

5. _____ is a decrease in the total amount of red blood cells (RBCs) or hemoglobin in the blood.

6. In medicine, _____ is a benign tumor occurring in areas lined with mucous membrane such as the nose, gastrointestinal tract, and the uterus.

7. _____ refers to bowel movements that are infrequent or hard to pass. The stool is often hard and dry.

8. The _____ tract is the tract from the mouth to the anus which includes all the organs of the digestive system in humans and other animals.

9. _____ cancer develops when tumorous growths develop in the large intestine. It is now the third most common type of cancer in the United States.

10. Her hands were misshapen by _____.

Ⅲ. Translation: translate the passage into Chinese.

Peptic ulcers are open sores that develop on the inside lining of your stomach and the upper portion of your small intestine. The most common symptom of a peptic ulcer is stomach pain. Peptic ulcers include gastric ulcers that occur on the inside of the stomach, duodenal ulcers that occur on the inside of the upper portion of your small intestine (duodenum). The most common causes of peptic ulcers are infection with the bacterium Helicobacter pylori (H. pylori) and long-term use of nonsteroidal anti-inflammatory drugs (NSAIDs) such as ibuprofen and naproxen sodium. Stress and spicy foods do not cause peptic ulcers. However, they can make your symptoms worse.

Peptic ulcers occur when acid in the digestive tract eats away at the inner surface of the stomach or small intestine. The acid can create a painful open sore that may bleed. Your digestive tract is coated with a mucous layer that normally protects against acid. But if the amount of acid is increased or the amount of mucus is decreased, you could develop an ulcer. Common causes include:

• A bacterium. Helicobacter pylori bacteria commonly live in the mucous layer that covers and protects tissues that line the stomach and small intestine. Often, the H. pylori bacterium causes no problems, but it can cause inflammation of the stomach's inner layer, producing an ulcer. It's not clear how H. pylori infection spreads. It may be transmitted from person to person by close contact, such as kissing. People may also contract H. pylori through food and water.

• Regular use of certain pain relievers. Taking aspirin, as well as certain over-the-counter and prescription pain medications called nonsteroidal anti-inflammatory drugs (NSAIDs), can irritate or inflame the lining of your stomach and small intestine. These medications include ibuprofen, naproxen sodium, ketoprofen and others. They do not include acetaminophen.

• Other medications. Taking certain other medications along with NSAIDs, such as steroids, anticoagulants, low-dose aspirin, selective serotonin reuptake inhibitors (SSRIs), alendronate and risedronate, can greatly increase the chance of developing ulcers.

(335 words)

IV. Give a presentation.

Dictate the causes, symptoms, treatments, etc. of Stomach Cancer in English with 3—4 students. Try to use the formal expression, especially related medical terminology when you make your presentation.

V. Write a birth certificate.

根据下列信息，撰写一份出生证明。

新生儿姓名：陈雯彰，女，2019 年 1 月 1 日 19 时 37 分出生于广东省妇幼保健院，39 孕周，3100 克，51 厘米，健康状况良好。母亲张洪，30 岁，汉族，身份证号：123456789654123624。父亲陈明涛，身份证号：125463217892125252，出生编号：12345。签发日期：2019 年 1 月 3 日。

Text B

Cirrhosis

Cirrhosis is a complication of many liver diseases characterized by abnormal structure and function of the liver. The diseases that lead to cirrhosis do so because they injure and kill liver cells, after which the inflammation and repair that is associated with the dying liver cells cause scar tissue to form. The liver cells that do not die multiply in an attempt to replace the cells that have died. This results in clusters of newly-formed liver cells within the scar tissue. There are many causes of cirrhosis including chemicals, viruses, toxic metals, and autoimmune liver disease in which the body's immune system attacks the liver.

Causes

Common causes of cirrhosis of the liver include:

- Alcohol;
- Nonalcoholic fatty liver disease;
- **Cryptogenic** causes;
- Chronic viral hepatitis (B, C, and D);
- Autoimmune hepatitis;
- Inherited (genetic) disorders;
- Primary **biliary** cirrhosis (PBC);
- Primary **sclerosing cholangitis** (PSC);
- Infants born without bile ducts.

Less common causes of cirrhosis include:

- Unusual reactions to some drugs;
- Prolonged exposure to toxins;
- Chronic heart failure (cardiac cirrhosis).

In certain parts of the world (particularly Northern Africa), infection of the liver with a **parasite (schistosomiasis)** is the most common cause of liver disease and cirrhosis.

Signs and symptoms

People with cirrhosis may have few or no symptoms and signs of liver disease. Common symptoms and signs of cirrhosis include:

- Yellowing of the skin (jaundice) due to the accumulation of **bilirubin** in the blood;
- Fatigue;
- Weakness;
- Loss of appetite;
- Itching;
- Easy bruising from decreased production of blood clotting factors by the diseased liver.

Stages

Cirrhosis in itself is already a late stage of liver damage. In the early stages of liver disease there will be inflammation of the liver. If this inflammation is not treated, it can lead to scarring (fibrosis). At this stage it is still possible for the liver to heal with treatment.

If fibrosis of the liver is not treated, it can result in cirrhosis. At this stage, the scar tissue cannot heal, but the progression of the scarring may be prevented or slowed. People with cirrhosis who have signs of complications may develop end-stage liver disease (ESLD) and the only treatment at this stage is liver transplantation.

- *Stage 1 cirrhosis* involves some scarring of the liver, but few symptoms. This stage is considered compensated cirrhosis, where there are no complications.
- *Stage 2 cirrhosis* includes worsening portal hypertension and the development of **varices**.
- *Stage 3 cirrhosis* involves the development of swelling in the abdomen and advanced liver scarring. This stage marks **decompensated** cirrhosis, with serious complications and possible liver failure.
- *Stage 4 cirrhosis* can be life threatening and people have develop end-stage liver disease (ESLD), which is fatal without a transplant.

Diagnosis and evaluation

The single best test for diagnosing cirrhosis is a biopsy of the liver. The history, physical examination, or routine testing may suggest the possibility of cirrhosis. If cirrhosis is present, other tests can be used to determine the severity of the cirrhosis and the presence of complications. Tests also may be used to diagnose the underlying disease that is causing the cirrhosis.

Examples of how doctors diagnose and evaluate cirrhosis are:

• The patient's history. A history of excessive and prolonged intake of alcohol, a history of intravenous drug abuse, or a history of hepatitis can suggest the possibility of liver disease and cirrhosis.

• Patients who are known to have chronic viral hepatitis B or C have a higher probability of having cirrhosis.

• Some patients with cirrhosis have enlarged livers and/or spleens.

• Some patients with cirrhosis, particularly alcoholic cirrhosis, have small red spider-like markings (**telangiectasias**) on the skin, particularly on the chest. However, these spider telangiectasias also can be seen in individuals without liver disease.

• Jaundice is common among patients with cirrhosis, but jaundice can occur in patients with liver diseases without cirrhosis and other conditions such as **hemolysis**.

• Swelling of the abdomen (**ascites**) and/or the lower extremities (**edema**) due to **retention** of fluid is common among patients with cirrhosis, although other diseases can cause them commonly.

• Patients with abnormal copper deposits in their eyes or certain types of neurologic disease may have Wilson disease, which can lead to cirrhosis.

• Esophageal varices may be found unexpectedly during upper endoscopy (EGD), strongly suggesting cirrhosis.

• Computerized **tomography** (CT or CAT) or magnetic resonance imaging (MRI) scans and ultrasound examinations of the abdomen done for reasons other than evaluating the possibility of liver disease may unexpectedly detect enlarged livers, abnormally **nodular** livers, enlarged spleens, and fluid in the abdomen, which suggest cirrhosis.

• Advanced cirrhosis leads to a reduced level of **albumin** in the blood and reduced blood clotting factors due to the loss of the liver's ability to produce these proteins. Reduced levels of albumin in the blood or abnormal bleeding suggest cirrhosis.

• An abnormal elevation of liver enzymes in the blood that are obtained routinely as part of yearly health examinations suggests inflammation or injury to the liver from many causes as well as cirrhosis.

• Patients with elevated levels of iron in their blood may have **hemochromatosis**, a genetic disease of the liver in which iron is handled abnormally and which leads to cirrhosis.

• Autoantibodies sometimes are detected in the blood and maybe a clue to the presence of autoimmune hepatitis or primary biliary cirrhosis, both of which can lead to cirrhosis.

- Liver cancer may be detected by CT and MRI scans or ultrasound of the abdomen. Liver cancer most commonly develops in individuals with underlying cirrhosis.
- Elevation of tumor markers such as alpha-fetoprotein suggests the presence of liver cancer.
- If there is an accumulation of fluid in the abdomen, a sample of the fluid can be removed using a long needle to be examined and tested. The results of testing may suggest the presence of cirrhosis as the cause of the fluid.

Treatment options

Preventing further damage to the liver
- Consume a balanced diet and one multivitamin daily.
- Avoid drugs (including alcohol) that cause liver damage. All patients with cirrhosis should avoid alcohol.
- Avoid nonsteroidal anti-inflammatory drugs (NSAIDs, e.g., ibuprofen). Patients with cirrhosis can experience worsening of liver and kidney function with NSAIDs.
- Eradicate hepatitis B and hepatitis C virus by using anti-viral medications.
- Remove blood from patients with hemochromatosis to reduce the levels of iron and prevent further damage to the liver.
- Suppress the immune system with drugs to decrease inflammation of the liver in autoimmune hepatitis.
- Immunize patients with cirrhosis against infection with hepatitis A and B to prevent a serious deterioration in liver. There are currently no vaccines available for immunizing against hepatitis C.

Prevention and early detection of liver cancer
Several types of liver disease that cause cirrhosis (such as hepatitis B and C) are associated with a high incidence of liver cancer. It is useful to screen for liver cancer in patients with cirrhosis, as early surgical treatment or transplantation of the liver can cure the patient of cancer.

Liver transplantation
Cirrhosis is irreversible. When cirrhosis is far advanced, liver transplantation often is the only option for treatment. Recent advances in surgical transplantation and medications to prevent infection and rejection of the transplanted liver have greatly improved survival after transplantation. On average, more than 80% of patients who receive transplants are alive after five years.

(1237 words)

Vocabulary

cirrhosis [sə'rəʊsɪs] *n.* 硬化, [内科] 肝硬化

cryptogenic [ˌkrɪptə'dʒenɪk] *adj.* (疾病) 隐源性的, (尤指疾病) 来源不明的

biliary ['bɪliəri] *adj.* 胆的, 胆汁的

sclerosing [sklɪə'rəʊsɪŋ] *adj.* 致硬化的, 硬化型的

cholangitis [kəʊlæn'dʒaɪtɪs] *n.* 胆道炎, [内科] 胆管炎

parasite ['pærəsaɪt] *n.* 寄生虫

schistosomiasis [ˌʃɪstəsəʊ'maɪəsɪs] *n.* [内科] 血吸虫病

bilirubin [ˌbɪlɪ'ruːbɪn] *n.* [生化] 胆红素

varix ['veərɪks] *n.* (复 varices) 静脉曲张

decompensate [diː'kɒmpənseɪt] *v.* 代谢失调

telangiectasia [telˌændʒɪˌek'teɪʒə] *n.* 毛细管扩张 (= telangiectasis)

hemolysis [hɪ'mɒlɪsɪs] *n.* [生理] [免疫] 溶血 (现象), 血细胞溶解

ascites [ə'saɪtiːz] *n.* [临床] 腹水

edema [ɪ'diːmə] *n.* [病理] 水肿 (= oedema), 瘤腺体

retention [rɪ'tenʃn] *n.* 保留, 滞留, 闭尿

tomography [tə'mɒgrəfi] *n.* X 线断层摄影术

nodular ['nɒdjʊlə(r)] *adj.* 结节状的, 有结节的

albumin ['ælbjʊmɪn] *n.* [生化] 白蛋白, [生化] 清蛋白

hemochromatosis [ˌheməˌkrəʊmə'təʊsɪs] *n.* [皮肤] 血色沉着病

Exercises

Ⅰ. **Decide whether the following sentences are *True* or *False* according to the text.**

1. Among the causes of cirrhosis, alcohol and chronic viral hepatitis (B, C, and D) are the common ones.

2. When cirrhosis is far advanced, liver transplantation often is not the only option for treatment.

3. Jaundice only occur in patients with cirrhosis.

4. Cirrhosis is a complication of liver diseases that injure liver cells and cause scar tissue to form.

5. Common causes of cirrhosis of the liver include chronic viral hepatitis, autoimmune hepatitis, inherited disorders, primary biliary cirrhosis, and alcohol, etc.

6. Common symptoms and signs of cirrhosis include jaundice, fatigue, weakness, loss of appetite, itching and bruising.

7. Stage 2 cirrhosis involves the development of swelling in the abdomen and advanced liver scarring.

8. Biopsy of the liver is the single best test for diagnosing cirrhosis, and other test

may suggest the possibility of cirrhosis.

9. Patients who have chronic viral hepatitis B or C have a higher risk of having cirrhosis.

10. Patients with cirrhosis can experience improvement of liver and kidney function with NSAIDs.

II. Fill in the blanks with the proper form of words in the box.

| jaundice | fibrosis | cirrhosis | ascites | varix | cholangitis |
| edema | hemolysis | decompensate | | telangiectasia | |

1. _____ is a chronic degenerative disease in which normal liver cells are damaged and are then replaced by scar tissue.

2. Mild _____ in the newborn is common and often clears without treatment.

3. Cystic _____ is an inherited disease characterized by the buildup of thick, sticky mucus that can damage many of the body's organs.

4. _____ is the abnormal buildup of fluid in the abdomen.

5. _____ refers to inflammation of the bile ducts owing to infection.

6. A _____ (pl. varices) is an abnormally dilated vessel with a tortuous course.

7. In medicine, _____ is the functional deterioration of a structure or system that had been previously working with the help of allostatic compensation.

8. _____ are small dilated blood vessels that can occur near the surface of the skin or mucous membrane.

9. _____ is the rupturing of red blood cells and the release of their contents into surrounding fluid.

10. _____ is the buildup of fluid in the body's tissue. Most commonly, the legs or arms are affected.

III. Translation: translate the passage into Chinese.

Viral hepatitis, mainly including hepatitis A, hepatitis B, and hepatitis C, are a group of distinct diseases that affect the liver. Some causes of hepatitis include prescription medications. Laboratory tests can determine hepatitis types.

What Is Hepatitis A?

Hepatitis A, also called hep A, is a contagious liver infection caused by the hepatitis A virus. Some people have only a mild illness that lasts a few weeks. Others have more severe problems that can last months. You usually get the disease when you eat or drink something contaminated by poop from a person who has the virus. The hepatitis A virus usually isn't dangerous. Almost everyone who has it gets better. But because it can take a while to go away, you'll need to take care of yourself in the meantime.

What Is Hepatitis B?

Hepatitis B is an infection of your liver. It's caused by a virus. There is a vaccine that protects against it. For some people, hepatitis B is mild and lasts a short time. These "acute" cases don't always need treatment. But it can become chronic. If that happens, it can cause scarring of the organ, liver failure, and cancer, and it even can be life-threatening. It's spread when people come in contact with the blood, open sores, or body fluids of someone who has the hepatitis B virus. It's serious, but if you get the disease as an adult, it shouldn't last a long time. Your body fights it off within a few months, and you're immune for the rest of your life. That means you can't get it again. But if you get it at birth, it's unlikely to go away.

What Is Hepatitis C?

Hepatitis C is a liver infection that can lead to serious liver damage. It's caused by the hepatitis C virus. About 3.9 million people in the U.S. have the disease. But it causes few symptoms, so most of them don't know. The virus spreads through an infected person's blood or body fluids. There are many forms of the hepatitis C virus, or HCV. The most common in the U.S. is type 1. Different forms of hepatitis C virus respond differently to treatment.

（385 words）

Ⅳ. **Give a presentation.**

Dictate the causes, symptoms, treatments, etc. of Cirrhosis in English with 3—4 students. Try to use the formal expression, especially related medical terminology when you make your presentation.

Ⅳ. **Write a death certificate.**

根据下列信息，写一份死亡证明。

患者 Allen Smith，男，87 岁，肝癌，于 2019 年 10 月 24 日在纽约 Memorial Sloan-Kettering 癌症中心过世。法院书记官是 Robbie James，副书记官是 Amanda Jones。

Text C

Colon Cancer

Colon cancer is a type of cancer that begins in the large intestine (colon). The colon is the final part of the digestive tract. Colon cancer typically affects older adults, though it can happen at any age. It usually begins as small, noncancerous (benign) clumps of cells called polyps that form on the inside of the colon. Over time some of these polyps can become colon cancers. Polyps may be small and produce few, if any, symptoms. For this reason, doctors recommend regular screening tests to help prevent colon cancer by identifying and removing polyps before they turn into cancer.

If colon cancer develops, many treatments are available to help control it, including surgery, radiation therapy and drug treatments, such as chemotherapy, targeted therapy and **immunotherapy**. Colon cancer is sometimes called **colorectal** cancer, which is a term that combines colon cancer and **rectal** cancer, which begins in the rectum.

Symptoms

Signs and symptoms of colon cancer include:

- A persistent change in your bowel habits, including diarrhea or constipation or a change in the consistency of your stool;
- Rectal bleeding or blood in your stool;
- Persistent abdominal discomfort, such as cramps, gas or pain;
- A feeling that your bowel doesn't empty completely;
- Weakness or fatigue;
- Unexplained weight loss.

Many people with colon cancer experience no symptoms in the early stages of the disease.

Causes

Doctors aren't certain what causes most colon cancers. In general, colon cancer begins when healthy cells in the colon develop changes (mutations) in their DNA. A cell's DNA contains a set of instructions that tell a cell what to do.

Healthy cells grow and divide in an orderly way to keep your body functioning normally. But when a cell's DNA is damaged and becomes cancerous, cells continue to divide—even when new cells aren't needed. As the cells accumulate, they form a tumor.

With time, the cancer cells can grow to invade and destroy normal tissue nearby. And cancerous cells can travel to other parts of the body to form deposits there (**metastasis**).

Diagnosis

If your signs and symptoms indicate that you could have colon cancer, your doctor may recommend one or more tests and procedures, including:

• Using a scope to examine the inside of your colon (colonoscopy). Colonoscopy uses a long, flexible and slender tube attached to a video camera and monitor to view your entire colon and rectum. If any suspicious areas are found, your doctor can pass surgical tools through the tube to take tissue samples (biopsies) for analysis and remove polyps.

• Blood tests. No blood test can tell you if you have colon cancer. But your doctor may test your blood for clues about your overall health, such as kidney and liver function tests.

Treatment

Which treatments are most likely to help you depends on your particular situation, including the location of your cancer, its stage and your other health concerns. Treatment for colon cancer usually involves surgery to remove the cancer. Other treatments, such as radiation therapy and chemotherapy, might also be recommended.

Surgery for early-stage colon cancer
If your colon cancer is very small, your doctor may recommend aminimally invasive approach to surgery, such as:

• Removing polyps during a colonoscopy (polypectomy). If your cancer is small, localized, completely contained within a polyp and in a very early stage, your doctor may be able to remove it completely during a colonoscopy.

• Endoscopic **mucosal** resection. Larger polyps might be removed during colonoscopy using special tools to remove the polyp and a small amount of the inner lining of the colon in a procedure called an endoscopic mucosal resection.

• Minimally invasive surgery (laparoscopic surgery). Polyps that can't be removed during a colonoscopy may be removed using laparoscopic surgery. In this procedure, your surgeon performs the operation through several small **incisions** in your abdominal wall, inserting instruments with attached cameras that display your colon on a video monitor.

Surgery for more advanced colon cancer

If the cancer has grown into or through your colon, your surgeon may recommend:

• Partial **colectomy**. During this procedure, the surgeon removes the part of your colon that contains the cancer, along with a margin of normal tissue on either side of the cancer.

• Surgery to create a way for waste to leave your body. When it's not possible to reconnect the healthy portions of your colon or rectum, you may need an **ostomy**. This involves creating an opening in the wall of your abdomen from a portion of the remaining bowel for the elimination of stool into a bag that fits securely over the opening.

• Lymph node removal. Nearby lymph nodes are usually also removed during colon cancer surgery and tested for cancer.

Surgery for advanced cancer

If your cancer is very advanced or your overall health very poor, your surgeon may recommend an operation to relieve a blockage of your colon or other conditions in order to improve your symptoms.

Chemotherapy

Chemotherapy uses drugs to destroy cancer cells. Chemotherapy for colon cancer is usually given after surgery if the cancer is larger or has spread to the lymph nodes.

Radiation therapy

Radiation therapy uses powerful energy sources, such as X-rays and protons, to kill cancer cells. It might be used to shrink a large cancer before an operation so that it can be removed more easily. Sometimes radiation is combined with chemotherapy.

Targeted drug therapy

Targeted drug treatments focus on specific abnormalities present within cancer cells. By blocking these abnormalities, targeted drug treatments can cause cancer cells to die. Targeted drugs are usually combined with chemotherapy.

Immunotherapy

Immunotherapy is a drug treatment that uses your immune system to fight cancer. Your body's disease-fighting immune system may not attack your cancer because the cancer cells produce proteins that blind the immune system cells from recognizing the cancer cells. Immunotherapy works by interfering with that process.

*Supportive (**palliative**) care*

Palliative care is specialized medical care that focuses on providing relief from pain and other symptoms of a serious illness.

（1004 words）

◆ **Vocabulary**

colon cancer 结直肠癌

immunotherapy [ɪˈmjʊnəʊˈθerəpi] *n.* 免疫疗法

colorectal [kəʊləˈrekt(ə)l] *adj.* 结肠直肠的

rectal [ˈrektəl] *adj.* 直肠的

metastasis [məˈtæstəsɪs] *n.* [医] 转移,转移瘤;新陈代谢

mucosal [mjuːˈkəʊsəl] *adj.* 黏膜的

incision [ɪnˈsɪʒn] *n.* 切口;雕刻,切割,切开

colectomy [kəˈlektəmi] *n.* [外科] 结肠切除术

ostomy [ˈɒstəmi] *n.* [外科] 造瘘术,造口术

palliative [ˈpæliətɪv] *n.* 缓和剂,姑息治疗,保守疗法 *adj.* 减轻痛苦的,缓解的

Text D

Gastroesophageal Reflux Disease

Gastroesophageal reflux disease (GERD) occurs when stomach acid frequently flows back into the tube connecting your mouth and stomach (esophagus). This backwash (acid reflux) can irritate the lining of your esophagus. Many people experience acid reflux from time to time. GERD is mild acid reflux that occurs at least twice a week, or moderate to severe acid reflux that occurs at least once a week. Most people can manage the discomfort of GERD with lifestyle changes and over-the-counter medications. But some people with GERD may need stronger medications or surgery to ease symptoms.

Symptoms

Common signs and symptoms of GERD include:

• A burning sensation in your chest (heartburn), usually after eating, which might be worse at night;

• Chest pain;   • Difficulty swallowing;
• Regurgitation of food or sour liquid;
• Sensation of a lump in your throat.

If you have nighttime acid reflux, you might also experience:

• Chronic cough;   • **Laryngitis**;
• New or worsening asthma;   • Disrupted sleep.

Causes

GERD is caused by frequent acid reflux. When you swallow, a circular band of muscle around the bottom of your esophagus (lower esophageal **sphincter**) relaxes to allow food and liquid to flow into your stomach. Then the sphincter closes again. If the sphincter relaxes abnormally or weakens, stomach acid can flow back up into your esophagus. This constant backwash of acid irritates the lining of your esophagus, often causing it to become inflamed.

Diagnosis

Your doctor might be able to diagnose GERD based on a physical examination and history of your signs and symptoms. To confirm a diagnosis of GERD, or to check for complications, your doctor might recommend:

• Upper endoscopy. Your doctor inserts a thin, flexible tube equipped with a light and camera (endoscope) down your throat, to examine the inside of your esophagus and stomach. Test results can often be normal when reflux is present, but an endoscopy may detect inflammation of the esophagus (esophagitis) or other complications. An endoscopy can also be used to collect a sample of tissue (biopsy) to be tested for complications such as Barrett's esophagus.

• Ambulatory acid (pH) probe test. A monitor is placed in your esophagus to identify when, and for how long, stomach acid regurgitates there. The monitor connects to a small computer that you wear around your waist or with a strap over your shoulder. The monitor might be a thin, flexible tube (catheter) that's threaded through your nose into your esophagus, or a clip that's placed in your esophagus during an endoscopy and that gets passed into your stool after about two days.

• Esophageal **manometry**. This test measures the rhythmic muscle contractions in your esophagus when you swallow. Esophageal manometry also measures the coordination and force exerted by the muscles of your esophagus.

• X-ray of your upper digestive system. X-rays are taken after you drink a chalky liquid that coats and fills the inside lining of your digestive tract. The coating allows your doctor to see a silhouette of your esophagus, stomach and upper intestine. You may also be asked to swallow a barium pill that can help diagnose a narrowing of the esophagus that may interfere with swallowing.

Treatment

Your doctor is likely to recommend that you first try lifestyle modifications and over-the-counter medications. If you don't experience relief within a few weeks, your doctor might recommend prescription medication or surgery.

Over-the-counter medications
The options include:

• **Antacids** that neutralize stomach acid. Antacids, such as **Mylanta**, Rolaids and Tums, may provide quick relief. But antacids alone won't heal an inflamed esophagus damaged by stomach acid. Overuse of some antacids can cause side effects, such as diarrhea or sometimes kidney problems.

• Medications to reduce acid production. These medications—known as H-2-receptor blockers—include cimetidine (Tagamet HB), famotidine (Pepcid AC) and nizatidine (Axid AR). H-2-receptor blockers don't act as quickly as antacids, but they provide longer relief and may decrease acid production from the stomach for up to 12 hours. Stronger versions are available by prescription.

• Medications that block acid production and heal the esophagus. These medications—known as proton pump inhibitors—are stronger acid blockers than H-2-receptor blockers and allow time for damaged esophageal tissue to heal. Over-the-counter proton pump inhibitors include **lansoprazole** (Prevacid 24 HR) and omeprazole (Prilosec OTC, Zegerid OTC).

Prescription medications

Prescription-strength treatments for GERD include:

• Prescription-strength H-2-receptor blockers. These include prescription-strength famotidine (Pepcid) and nizatidine. These medications are generally well-tolerated but long-term use may be associated with a slight increase in risk of vitamin B_{12} deficiency and bone fractures.

• Prescription-strength proton pump inhibitors. These include **esomeprazole** (Nexium), lansoprazole (Prevacid), omeprazole (Prilosec, Zegerid), pantoprazole (Protonix), **rabeprazole** (Aciphex) and **Dexlansoprazole** (Dexilant). Although generally well-tolerated, these medications might cause diarrhea, headache, nausea and vitamin B_{12} deficiency. Chronic use might increase the risk of hip fracture.

• Medication to strengthen the lower esophageal sphincter. Baclofen may ease GERD by decreasing the frequency of relaxations of the lower esophageal sphincter. Side effects might include fatigue or nausea.

Surgery and other procedures

GERD can usually be controlled with medication. But if medications don't help or you wish to avoid long-term medication use, your doctor might recommend:

• **Fundoplication**. The surgeon wraps the top of your stomach around the lower esophageal sphincter, to tighten the muscle and prevent reflux. Fundoplication is usually done with a minimally invasive (laparoscopic) procedure. The wrapping of the top part of the stomach can be partial or complete.

• LINX device. A ring of tiny magnetic beads is wrapped around the junction of the stomach and esophagus. The magnetic attraction between the beads is strong enough to keep the junction closed to refluxing acid, but weak enough to allow food to pass through. The LINX device can be implanted using minimally invasive surgery.

• **Transoral** incisionless fundoplication (TIF). This new procedure involves tightening the lower esophageal sphincter by creating a partial wrap around the lower esophagus using polypropylene fasteners. TIF is performed through the mouth with a device called an endoscope and requires no surgical incision. Its advantages include quick recovery time and high tolerance.

If you have a large **hiatal hernia**, TIF alone is not an option. However, it may be possible if TIF is combined with laparoscopic hiatal hernia repair.

Lifestyle and home remedies

Lifestyle changes may help reduce the frequency of acid reflux. Try to:

• Maintain a healthy weight.
• Stop smoking.
• Elevate the head of your bed. If you regularly experience heartburn while trying to sleep, place wood or cement blocks under the feet of your bed so that the head end is raised by 6 to 9 inches.
• Don't lie down after a meal. Wait at least three hours after eating before lying down or going to bed.
• Eat food slowly and chew thoroughly. Put down your fork after every bite and pick it up again once you have chewed and swallowed that bite.
• Avoid foods and drinks that trigger reflux.
• Avoid tight-fitting clothing. Clothes that fit tightly around your waist put pressure on your abdomen and the lower esophageal sphincter.

（1179 words）

◆ **Vocabulary**

gastroesophageal reflux disease 胃食管反流病

laryngitis［ˌlærɪnˈdʒaɪtɪs］*n.*［耳鼻喉］喉炎

sphincter［ˈsfɪŋktə(r)］*n.*［解剖］括约肌

manometry［məˈnɒmɪtri］*n.* 测压法

antacid［æntˈæsɪd］*n.* 抗酸剂，解酸药
　adj. 中和酸的

mylanta *n.* 碳酸钙制剂（抗酸药），胃能达

lansoprazole 南索拉唑，兰索拉唑

esomeprazole［ˈesəmprəzəul］埃索美拉唑，

艾司奥美拉唑

rabeprazole［rəbprəˈzəul］［医］雷贝拉唑（抗溃疡药）

Dexlansoprazole 右兰索拉唑

fundoplication［fʌnˈdɒplɪkeɪʃn］胃底折叠术，胃底折术

transoral 经口的

hiatal［haɪˈeɪtəl］*adj.* 裂孔的，空隙的

hiatal hernia［内科］食管裂孔疝

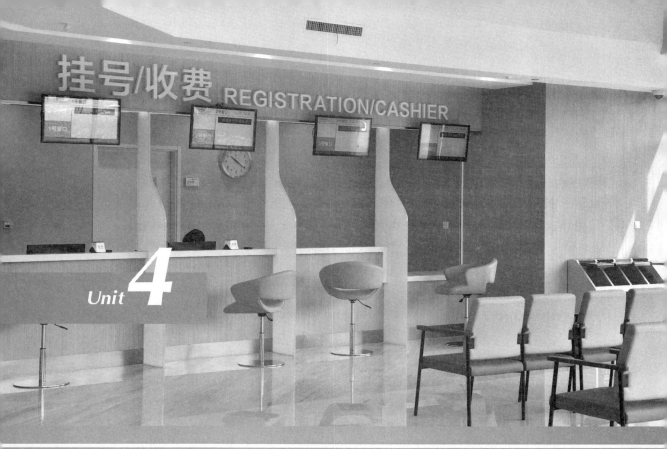

Unit 4

Some Common Diseases of the Urinary System

✓参考答案
✓微课等资源

Text A

Cystitis

Cystitis is a fairly common lower urinary tract infection. It refers specifically to an inflammation of the bladder wall. Although cystitis is not normally a serious condition, it can be uncomfortable and lead to complications if left untreated.

Facts

- Cystitis is most commonly caused by a bacterial infection.
- In most cases, mild cystitis will resolve itself within a few days.
- If it persists for more than 4 days, it should be discussed with a doctor.

Cystitis usually occurs when the urethra and bladder, which are normally **sterile**, or microbe-free, become infected with bacteria. Bacteria fasten to the lining of the bladder and cause the area to become irritated and inflamed. Cystitis affects people of both sexes and all ages. It is more common among females than males because women have shorter urethras. Around 80 percent of all urinary tract infections (UTIs) are caused by bacteria from the bowel that reach the urinary tract. Most of these bacteria form part of the healthy **intestinal flora**, but once they enter the sterile space in the urethra and bladder, they can cause a UTI. UTIs are the most common **hospital-acquired infections** in the United States, especially among patients using urinary catheters.

Symptoms

The following are common signs and symptoms of cystitis:

- Traces of blood in the urine;
- Dark, cloudy, or strong-smelling urine;
- Pain just above the **pubic bone**, in the lower back, or in the abdomen;
- Burning sensation when urinating;
- Urinating frequently or feeling the need to urinate frequently.

Elderly individuals may feel weak and feverish but have none of the other symptoms mentioned above. They may also present with altered mental status. There is a frequent need to urinate, but only small amounts of urine are passed each time.

When children have cystitis, they may have any of the symptoms listed above, plus vomiting and general weakness.

Some other illnesses or conditions have similar symptoms to cystitis, and these include:

- **Urethritis**, or inflammation of the urethra;
- Bladder pain syndrome;
- **Prostatitis**, or inflammation of the **prostate** gland;
- Benign prostatic **hyperplasia**, in men;
- Lower urinary tract syndrome;
- **Gonorrhea**;
- **Chlamydia**;
- **Candida**, or **thrush**.

Causes

There are many possible causes of cystitis. Most are infectious, and the majority of these cases stem from an **ascending infection**. The bacteria enter from the external **genitourinary** structures.

Risk factors

- **Tampon** use: When inserting a tampon, there is a slight risk of bacteria entering via the urethra.
- Inserting, changing, or prolonged use of a urinary catheter. There is a chance the catheter will carry bacteria along the urinary tract.
- **Diaphragm** for birth control: There is a higher incidence of cystitis among women who use the diaphragm with **spermicides**, compared with sexually active women who do not use one.
- Full bladder: If the bladder is not emptied completely, it creates an environment for bacteria to multiply. This is fairly common among pregnant women or men whose prostates are enlarged.
- Sexual activity: Sexually active women have a higher risk of bacteria entering via the urethra.
- Blockage in part of the urinary system that prevents the flow of urine.
- Other bladder or kidney problems.
- Frequent or vigorous sex: This increases the chances of physical damage, which in turn increases the likelihood of cystitis. This is sometimes

called honeymoon cystitis.

• Falling **estrogen** levels: During menopause, estrogen levels drop, and the lining of a woman's urethra gets thinner. The thinner the lining becomes, the higher the chances are of infection and damage. After menopause, the risk is higher.

• Gender: A woman's urethra opening is nearer the **anus** than a man's, so there is a higher risk of bacteria from the intestines entering the urethra.

• Mucus reduction: During menopause, women produce less mucus in the vaginal area. This mucus normally acts as a protective layer against bacteria.

• Radiotherapy: Damage to the bladder can cause late radiation cystitis.

Women on hormone replacement therapy (HRT) have a lower risk of developing cystitis compared with menopausal women not on HRT. However, HRT has its own set of risks, so it is not routinely used for the treatment of infectious cystitis in post-menopausal women.

Diagnosis

A doctor will ask the patient some questions, carry out an examination, and do a urine test. The urine test will either be sent to a laboratory, or the doctor may use a dipstick. Urine dipstick results come back quickly while the patient is still in the office.

A urine culture or catheterized urine specimen may be performed to determine the type of bacteria in the urine. After finding out which specific bacterium is causing the infection, the doctor will prescribe an oral antibiotic.

Most doctors will also offer to test for a sexually transmitted infection (STI). STIs often have similar symptoms to cystitis.

Patients who get cystitis regularly may need further tests. This could include an ultrasound scan, an X-ray, or a **cystoscopy** of the bladder, using a fiber-optic camera.

Remedies

The following home remedies and measures may help:

• Painkillers, such as acetaminophen (Tylenol) or ibuprofen, may relieve discomfort. These are available to purchase online.
• Water and other fluids help flush the bacteria through the system.
• Alcohol should be avoided.
• Cranberries contain an active ingredient that prevents bacteria from

sticking to the bladder wall, but **cranberry** juice or capsules may not contain enough active ingredient to prevent symptoms.

• Refraining from sex reduces the chance of bacteria entering the urethra.

Treatment

Most cases of mild cystitis will resolve itself within a few days. Any cystitis that lasts more than 4 days should be discussed with a doctor. Doctors may prescribe a 3-day or 7-10 day course of antibiotics, depending on the patient. This should start to ease symptoms within a day. If symptoms do not improve after taking the antibiotics, the patient should return to the doctor.

Antibiotics commonly used for bacterial cystitis are **nitrofurantoin**, **trimethoprim-sulfamethoxazole**, **amoxicillin**, **cephalosporins**, **ciprofloxacin**, and **levofloxacin**.

In older people and those with weakened immune systems, due, for example, to diabetes, have a higher risk of the infection spreading to the kidney and other complications. Vulnerable people and pregnant women should be treated promptly.

Prevention

Cystitis is often not preventable, but the following measures may help:

• Practicing good hygiene after sex.
• Using neutral, unperfumed soaps around the **genitals**. Soaps for sensitive skin are available to purchase online.
• Emptying the bladder completely when urinating.
• Not postponing urination.
• Avoiding tight underwear and tight pants.
• Wearing cotton underwear. Different styles are available to buy online.
• Wiping from front to back.
• Using a **lubricant** during sex. Compare different brands online before purchasing.

Those who use catheters should ask a doctor or nurse how to avoid damage when changing the catheter.

（1142 words）

◆ Vocabulary

cystitis [sɪˈstaɪtɪs] n. [泌尿] 膀胱炎

sterile [ˈsteraɪl] adj. 无菌的；不育的

flora [ˈflɔːrə] n. 菌群；植物群

intestinal flora [ɪnˈtestɪnl ˈflɔːrə] 肠菌类

hospital-acquired infection 医院感染

pubic [ˈpjuːbɪk] adj. 耻骨的；阴毛的，阴部的

pubic bone [解剖] 耻骨

urethritis [ˌjʊərəˈθraɪtɪs] n. [泌尿] 尿道炎

prostatitis [ˌprɒstəˈtaɪtɪs] n. [泌尿] 前列腺炎

prostate [ˈprɒsteɪt] n. 前列腺 adj. 前列腺的

hyperplasia [ˌhaɪpəˈpleɪʒə] n. [病理] 增生

gonorrhea [ɡɒnəˈriːə] n. [性病] 淋病

chlamydia [kləˈmɪdiə] n. 衣原体

candida [ˈkændɪdə] n. 念珠菌属，假丝酵母

thrush [θrʌʃ] n. [口腔] 鹅口疮

ascending infection 上行性感染

genitourinary [ˌdʒenɪtəʊˈjʊərɪnəri] adj. [解剖] 泌尿生殖器的

tampon [ˈtæmpən] n. 止血棉球；止血栓

diaphragm [ˈdaɪəfræm] n. 隔膜；子宫帽

spermicide [ˈspɜːmɪsaɪd] n. 杀精子剂

estrogen [ˈiːstrədʒən] n. 雌性激素

anus [ˈeɪnəs] n. [解剖] 肛门

cystoscopy [sɪsˈtɒskəpi] n. [泌尿] 膀胱镜检查

cranberry [ˈkrænbəri] n. 蔓越莓

nitrofurantoin [ˌnaɪtrəʊfjʊˈræntəɪn] n. 呋喃妥英

trimethoprim [traɪˈmeθəprɪm] n. [药] 甲氧苄啶

sulfamethoxazole [sʌlˈfæmtɒksəzəʊl] n. 磺胺甲恶唑

amoxicillin [əˈmɒksɪˌsɪlɪn] n. 阿莫西林，羟氨苄青霉素

cephalosporins [sefələʊsˈpɔːrɪnz] n. [药] 头孢霉菌素

ciprofloxacin [sɪprəʊˈflɒksəsɪn] n. 环丙沙星，环丙氟哌酸

levofloxacin [levəflɒkˈseɪsɪn] n. 左氧氟沙星

genital [ˈdʒenɪtl] n. 生殖器，外阴部 adj. 生殖的，生殖器的

lubricant [ˈluːbrɪkənt] n. 润滑剂，润滑油 adj. 润滑的

◆ Exercises

Ⅰ. **Decide whether the following sentences are *True* or *False* according to the text.**

1. Cystitis usually occurs when the urethra and bladder, which are normally sterile, or microbe-free, become infected with virus.

2. Children with cystitis have the same symptoms as older people.

3. If you have symptoms such as blood in the urine, strong-smelling urine and burning sensation, it means that you may have the disease of cystitis.

4. Possible causes of cystitis are many, but the most common one is bacterial

infection.

5. Cystitis is more common among females than males because women have shorter urethras.

6. Women with menopause develop higher risk factors of cystitis than women without menopause.

7. There is a chance that the use of a urinary catheter will carry bacteria along the urinary tract which is normally sterile, or microbe-free.

8. If you have cystitis, you can use alcohol for home remedy.

9. Wearing loose and cotton underwear is better than tight and nylon one to prevent cystitis.

10. Frequent sex has nothing to do with increasing the likelihood of cystitis.

Ⅱ. **Fill in the blanks with the proper form of words in the box.**

chlamydia	bowel	cystitis	urethritis	pubic
sterile	thrush	hyperplasia	prostatitis	gonorrhea

1. _____ is defined as inflammation of the urinary bladder.

2. He always made sure that any cuts were protected by _____ dressings.

3. The boy was suffering from a _____ obstruction.

4. In vertebrates, the _____ bone is the most forward-facing (ventral and anterior) of the three main bones making up the pelvis.

5. _____ is the inflammation of the urethra. The most common symptoms include painful or difficult urination and urethral discharge.

6. _____ is inflammation of the prostate gland.

7. _____ is an increase in the amount of organic tissue that results from cell proliferation.

8. _____ is a sexually transmitted infection (STI) caused by the bacterium Neisseria gonorrhoeae.

9. _____ is a sexually transmitted infection caused by the bacterium Chlamydia trachomatis.

10. _____ is infection of the oral mucous membrane by the fungus Candida albicans.

Ⅲ. **Translation: translate the passage into Chinese.**

A urinary tract infection (UTI) is an infection in any part of your urinary system—your kidneys, ureters, bladder and urethra. Most infections involve the lower urinary tract—the bladder and the urethra. Women are at greater risk of developing a UTI than men. Infection limited to your bladder can be painful and annoying. However, serious consequences can occur if a UTI spreads to your kidneys. Doctors typically treat urinary tract infections with antibiotics. But you can take steps to reduce your chances of getting a UTI in the first place.

Urinary tract infections typically occur when bacteria enter the urinary tract through the urethra and begin to multiply in the bladder. Although the urinary system is designed to keep out such microscopic invaders, these defenses sometimes fail. When that happens, bacteria may take hold and grow into a full-blown infection in the urinary tract. The most common UTIs occur mainly in women and affect the bladder and urethra.

- Infection of the bladder (cystitis). This type of UTI is usually caused by Escherichia coli (E. coli), a type of bacteria commonly found in the gastrointestinal (GI) tract. However, sometimes other bacteria are responsible. Sexual intercourse may lead to cystitis, but you don't have to be sexually active to develop it. All women are at risk of cystitis because of their anatomy—specifically, the short distance from the urethra to the anus and the urethral opening to the bladder.

- Infection of the urethra (urethritis). This type of UTI can occur when GI bacteria spread from the anus to the urethra. Also, because the female urethra is close to the vagina, sexually transmitted infections, such as herpes, gonorrhea, chlamydia and mycoplasma can cause urethritis.

(288 words)

Ⅳ. Give a presentation.

Dictate the causes, symptoms, treatments, etc. of Cystitis in English with 3—4 students. Try to use the formal expression, especially related medical terminology when you make your presentation.

Ⅴ. Write a certificate of hospital transfer.

根据下列内容,写一份转院证明。

王某,男,50 岁,患骨癌,需转至中山大学附属肿瘤医院做进一步检查和治疗。广东惠州人民医院主治医生李伟, 2019 年 3 月 3 日。

Text B

Nephritis

Nephritis is a condition in which the **nephrons**, the functional units of the kidneys, become inflamed. This inflammation, which is also known as **glomerulonephritis**, can adversely affect kidney function.

The kidneys are bean-shaped organs that filter the blood circulating the body to remove excess water and waste products from it.

There are many types of nephritis with a range of causes. While some types occur suddenly, others develop as part of a chronic condition and require ongoing management.

Types

There are several different types of nephritis, including:

Acute glomerulonephritis: This form of nephritis can develop suddenly after a severe infection, such as strep throat, hepatitis, or HIV. Lupus and rarer disorders, such as **vasculitides** and **granulomatosis** with polyangiitis (GPA), can also lead to acute inflammation of the kidneys. A person with these conditions will require prompt medical attention during a flare-up to reduce kidney damage.

Lupus nephritis: Lupus is an autoimmune disease, which means that the immune system mistakenly attacks healthy tissues in the body. Over half of all individuals with a lupus diagnosis eventually develop lupus nephritis. This occurs when the immune system attacks the kidneys. The symptoms of lupus nephritis include:

- **Foamy** urine;
- High blood pressure;
- Swelling of the legs, ankles, and feet.

People may also notice symptoms in other parts of the body. These symptoms may include joint problems, fever, and rashes. The severity of lupus can vary between patients. Although the disease sometimes goes into **remission**, the condition can become serious. It is vital for anyone experiencing symptoms of lupus nephritis to seek prompt medical attention to limit further kidney damage.

Alport syndrome, or *hereditary nephritis*: This disease can lead to kidney failure, as well as vision and hearing problems. Alport syndrome is passed on in the genes, and it is usually more severe in men.

Chronic glomerulonephritis: This form of nephritis develops slowly and causes few symptoms in its early stages. As with acute glomerulonephritis, this condition can cause severe kidney damage and kidney failure. It may run in families or develop after a sudden disease.

IgA nephropathy: This is one of the more common forms of nephritis. It develops when IgA antibody deposits build up in the kidneys and cause inflammation. The immune system develops antibodies to combat harmful substances and organisms that enter the body. People with IgA neuropathy have defective IgA antibodies. Doctors do not often find IgA nephropathy in young people, as the early symptoms are easy to miss. People can treat this condition with blood pressure medications.

Interstitial nephritis: Often developing very rapidly, this form of nephritis usually occurs due to infection or a particular medication. It affects the part of the kidney called the **interstitium**, which is a fluid-filled space.

If a doctor takes the affected individual off the problematic medication quickly, a full recovery is possible in a few weeks. However, damage can sometimes accumulate to the point of kidney failure.

Causes

There are many different causes of nephritis. In some cases, the cause may not be clear. Nephritis and kidney disease often seem to run in families, which suggests a possible genetic component. Some infections, such as HIV and hepatitis B or C, can also cause nephritis. In some cases, kidney damage can occur as a result of medications, such as antibiotics. This damage can lead to nephritis. Taking too many pain relievers, nonsteroidal anti-inflammatory drugs (NSAIDs), or diuretic pills can also cause this condition.

Anatomy of the kidneys

The two kidneys are bean-shaped, fist-sized organs that sit just beneath the ribs on either side of the **spine**. They remove impurities and extra water from the blood, filtering about 150 quarts of blood a day.

Each kidney consists of thousands of structures called nephrons, in which the blood filtering takes place. In each nephron, a two-step cleaning process separates necessary nutrients from waste products. A filter called the

glomerulus catches blood cells and protein, sending water and waste to a second filter, called a **tubule**. The tubule captures minerals and extra protein. After that, waste materials leave the body in the urine.

In people with nephritis, both the tubules and nearby tissues become inflamed, which can lead to kidney damage. Damaged kidneys are unable to function at full capacity. Waste builds up and causes serious health problems. If the condition is severe or persistent enough, it can result in kidney failure.

Risk factors

The most important risk factors for kidney disease are:

- A family history of kidney disease;
- High blood pressure;
- Diabetes;
- Obesity;
- Heart disease;
- An age of 60 years or more.

Symptoms

The symptoms of nephritis are rarely severe in the early stages. The following signs may indicate that a person has this condition:

- Changes in urinating habits;
- Swelling anywhere in the body, especially the hands, feet, ankles, and face;
- Changes in urine color;
- Foamy urine;
- Blood in the urine.

When to see a doctor

Urine that contains blood will appear brown or pink. Anyone with this sign should visit a doctor as soon as possible. It is also best to seek medical attention for any other symptoms involving the urine. Early treatment can prevent permanent kidney damage and the more severe complications of nephritis.

Diagnosis

In some cases, a doctor may detect nephritis during a routine blood or urine test. Finding protein in the urine can indicate that the kidneys are not working correctly. A blood test that measures a waste product in the blood called **creatinine** can also provide information on the health of the kidneys. However, a biopsy is the best way to check for nephritis. For this procedure, a doctor will remove a piece of the kidney with a needle and send it to a laboratory for analysis.

Treatment

The treatment for nephritis may vary according to the cause and type.

Acute nephritis sometimes resolves without treatment. However, it usually requires medication and special procedures that remove excess fluids and dangerous proteins. Treating chronic nephritis typically involves regular kidney check-ups and blood pressure monitoring. Doctors may prescribe water pills to control blood pressure and reduce any swelling. Medications that prevent the immune system from attacking the kidneys can also be beneficial in some cases.

Doctors may also refer an individual with kidney infection to a **dietitian**, who can advise them on what to eat to protect their kidneys. A suitable diet will typically be lower in protein, salt, and **potassium**.

Prevention

Although it is not always possible to prevent nephritis, certain lifestyle practices can reduce the risk for many people. These practices include:

- Maintaining a healthy weight;
- Quitting smoking;
- Keeping blood pressure and blood sugar within healthy limits;
- Exercising regularly;
- Eating a nutritious, balanced diet can also help protect kidney health.

（1127 words）

◆ Vocabulary

nephritis [nɪˈfraɪtɪs] n. ［泌尿］肾炎 (复数 nephritides)

nephron [ˈnefrɒn] n. ［解剖］肾单位，肾元

glomerulonephritis [ˌglɒmerjuːləʊnefˈraɪtɪs] n. ［泌尿］肾小球性肾炎

vasculitides [ˌvaskjuˈlɪtɪdiːz] n. 血管炎

granulomatosis [ˌgrænjuləʊməˈtəʊsɪs] n. 肉芽肿性疾病

lupus nephritis ［内科］狼疮性肾炎

foamy [ˈfəʊmi] adj. 起泡沫的，布满泡沫的，泡沫似的

remission [rɪˈmɪʃn] n. 缓解；宽恕

Alport syndrome 奥尔波特综合征
hereditary nephritis 遗传性肾炎
nephropathy [nə'frɒpəθi] n. 肾病
interstitial nephritis 间质性肾炎
interstitium [ɪntəs'tɪʃəm] n. 小间隙
spine [spaɪn] n. 脊柱，脊椎

glomerulus [glɒ'merjʊləs] n. 肾小球
tubule ['tjuːbjuːl] n.小管，细管
creatinine [kri:'ætiniːn] n. [生化]肌酸酐
dietitian [ˌdaɪə'tɪʃn] n.营养学家，饮食学家
potassium [pə'tæsiəm] n. [化学]钾

◇ Exercises

Ⅰ. **Decide whether the following sentences are *True* or *False* according to the text.**

1. The kidneys are bean-shaped organs that filter the blood to remove excess water and waste products from it.

2. Lupus nephritis is a disease, which means that the immune system can not mistakenly attacks healthy tissues in the body.

3. Nephritis and kidney disease often seem to run in families, which suggests a possible genetic component.

4. Generally speaking, HIV and hepatitis B or C can not cause nephritis.

5. Heart disease and diabetes are not risk factors for nephritis.

6. In each nephron, a two-step cleaning process separates necessary nutrients from waste products. One is glomerulus and the other is tubule.

7. Foamy urine and blood in the urine are symptoms of nephritis, but changes in urine color is not a symptom of the disease.

8. Doctors often find IgA nephropathy in young people, as the early symptoms are easy to find.

9. IgA nephropathy can lead to kidney failure, as well as vision and hearing problems.

10. Interstitial nephritis often develops very rapidly, and this form of nephritis usually occurs due to infection or a particular medication.

Ⅱ. **Fill in the blanks with the proper form of words in the box.**

nephritis	mimicking	spine	tubule	glomerulus
dialysis	lupus	nephropathy	dietitian	vasculitides

1. The computer doesn't _____ human thought, but it reaches the same ends by different means.

2. He was on _____ for seven years before his first kidney transplant.

3. The _____ was helpful, making suggestions as to how I could improve

my diet.

4. In biology, a _____ is a general term referring to small tube or similar type of structure.

5. The _____ is an integral part of the nephron, the basic unit of the kidney.

6. _____ is the main part of the axial skeleton of vertebrate animals and of man.

7. _____ is damage to or disease of a kidney.

8. _____ is the inflammation of a blood vessel or a lymph vessel.

9. _____ is an autoimmune disease in which the body's immune system mistakenly attacks healthy tissue in many parts of the body.

10. _____ is inflammation of the kidneys and may involve the glomeruli, tubules, or interstitial tissue surrounding the glomeruli and tubules.

Ⅲ. Translation: translate the passage into Chinese.

A kidney transplant is a surgical procedure to place a healthy kidney from a living or deceased donor into a person whose kidneys no longer function properly.

When your kidneys lose this filtering ability, harmful levels of fluid and waste accumulate in your body, which can raise your blood pressure and result in kidney failure (end-stage kidney disease). End-stage renal disease occurs when the kidneys have lost about 90% of their ability to function normally. Common causes of end-stage kidney disease include diabetes, chronic, uncontrolled high blood pressure, chronic glomerulonephritis—an inflammation and eventual scarring of the tiny filters within your kidneys (glomeruli), and polycystic kidney disease. People with end-stage renal disease need to have waste removed from their bloodstream via a machine (dialysis) or a kidney transplant to stay alive.

If a compatible living donor isn't available, your name may be placed on a kidney transplant waiting list to receive a kidney from a deceased donor. How long you have to wait for a deceased donor organ depends on the degree of matching or compatibility between you and the donor, time on dialysis and on the transplant waitlist, and expected survival post-transplant. Some people get a match within several months, and others may wait several years.

Kidney transplantation can treat advanced kidney disease and kidney failure, but it is not a cure. Some forms of kidney disease may return after transplant. The health risks associated with kidney transplant include those associated directly with the surgery itself, rejection of the donor organ and side effects of taking medications (anti-rejection or immunosuppressants) needed to prevent your body from rejecting the donated kidney.

Deciding whether kidney transplant is right for you is a personal decision that deserves careful thought and consideration of the serious risks and benefits. Talk through your decision with your friends, family and other trusted advisors.

After a successful kidney transplant, your new kidney will filter your blood, and you will no longer need dialysis. To prevent your body from rejecting your donor kidney, you'll need medications to suppress your immune system. Because these anti-rejection medications make your body more vulnerable to infection, your doctor may also prescribe antibacterial, antiviral and antifungal medications. It is important to take all your medicines as your doctor prescribes. Your body may reject your new kidney if you skip your medications even for a short period of time.

(396 words)

IV. Give a presentation.

Dictate the causes, symptoms, treatments, etc. of Nephritis in English with 3—4 students. Try to use the formal expression, especially related medical terminology when you make your presentation.

V. Write a certificate of discharge.

根据下列内容,写一份出院证明。

李某,女,35 岁,因患急性阑尾炎于 2022 年 3 月 20 日入院治疗。经两周的治疗,现已痊愈,将于 2022 年 4 月 6 日出院。其健康状况良好,休息 3 天后可恢复工作。必要时,来医院检查。广州市红十字会医院主治医生刘明,2022 年 4 月 5 日。

Text C

Diabetic Nephropathy

Diabetic nephropathy is a serious kidney-related complication of type 1 diabetes and type 2 diabetes. It is also called diabetic kidney disease. About 25% of people with diabetes eventually develop kidney disease. Diabetic nephropathy affects your kidneys' ability to do their usual work of removing waste products and extra fluid from your body. The best way to prevent or delay diabetic nephropathy is by maintaining a healthy lifestyle and treating your diabetes and high blood pressure. Over many years, the condition slowly damages your kidneys' delicate filtering system. Early treatment may prevent or slow the disease's progress and reduce the chance of complications.

Your kidney disease may progress to kidney failure, also called end-stage kidney disease. Kidney failure is a life-threatening condition. At this stage your treatment options are dialysis or a kidney transplant.

Symptoms

In the early stages of diabetic nephropathy, you may not notice any signs or symptoms. In later stages, the signs and symptoms include:

- Worsening blood pressure control;
- Protein in the urine;
- Swelling of feet, ankles, hands or eyes;
- Increased need to urinate;
- Reduced need for **insulin** or diabetes medicine;
- Confusion or difficulty concentrating;
- Shortness of breath;
- Loss of appetite;
- Nausea and vomiting;
- Persistent itching;
- Fatigue.

Causes

Diabetic nephropathy results when diabetes damages blood vessels and other cells in your kidneys.

How the kidneys work

Your kidneys contain millions of tiny blood vessel clusters (**glomeruli**) that filter waste from your blood. Severe damage to these blood vessels can lead to diabetic nephropathy, decreased kidney function and kidney failure.

Diabetic nephropathy causes

Diabetic nephropathy is a common complication of type 1 and type 2 diabetes.

Over time, poorly controlled diabetes can cause damage to blood vessel clusters in your kidneys that filter waste from your blood. This can lead to kidney damage and cause high blood pressure. High blood pressure can cause further kidney damage by increasing the pressure in the delicate filtering system of the kidneys.

Diagnosis

Your doctor will ask you about your signs and symptoms, conduct a physical exam, and ask about your medical history. He or she may refer you to a kidney specialist (**nephrologist**) or a diabetes specialist (**endocrinologist**). To determine whether you have diabetic kidney disease, you may need certain tests and procedures, such as:

• Blood tests. If you have diabetes, you will need blood tests to monitor your condition and determine how well your kidneys are working.

• Urine tests. Urine samples provide information about your kidney function and whether you have too much protein in the urine. High levels of a protein called **microalbumin** may indicate your kidneys are being affected by disease.

• Imaging tests. Your doctor may use X-rays and ultrasound to assess your kidneys' structure and size. You may also undergo CT scanning and magnetic resonance imaging (MRI) to determine how well blood is circulating within your kidneys. Other imaging tests may be used in some cases.

• Renal function testing. Your doctor can assess your kidneys' filtering capacity using renal analysis testing.

• Kidney biopsy. Your doctor may recommend a kidney biopsy to remove a sample of kidney tissue. You'll be given a numbing medication (local anesthetic). Then your doctor will use a thin needle to remove small pieces of kidney tissue for examination under a microscope.

Treatment

The first step in treating diabetic nephropathy is to treat and control your diabetes and, if needed, high blood pressure (hypertension). With good management of your blood sugar and hypertension, you can prevent or delay kidney dysfunction and other complications.

Medications

In the early stages of the disease, your treatment plan may include various medications, such as those that help:

• Control high blood pressure. Medications called angiotensin-converting enzyme (ACE) **inhibitors** and angiotensin II receptor blockers (ARBs) are used to treat high blood pressure. Using both of these together isn't advised because of increased side effects. Studies support the goal of a blood pressure reading below 140/90 millimeters of **mercury** (mm Hg) depending on your age and overall risk of cardiovascular disease.

• Manage high blood sugar. Several medications have been shown to help control high blood sugar in people with diabetic nephropathy. Studies support the goal of an average **hemoglobin** A1C of less than 7%.

• Lower high cholesterol. Cholesterol-lowering drugs called statins are used to treat high cholesterol and reduce protein in the urine.

• Foster bone health. Medications that help manage your calcium **phosphate** balance are important in maintaining healthy bones.

• Control protein in urine. Medications can often reduce the level of the protein albumin in the urine and improve kidney function.

Your doctor may recommend follow-up testing at regular intervals to see whether your kidney disease remains stable or progresses.

Treatment for advanced diabetic kidney disease

If your disease progresses to kidney failure (end-stage kidney disease), your doctor will help you transition to care focused on either replacing the function of your kidneys or making you more comfortable. Options include:

• Kidney dialysis. This treatment is a way to remove waste products and extra fluid from your blood. The two main types of dialysis are **hemodialysis** and **peritoneal** dialysis. In the first, more common method, you may need to visit a dialysis center and be connected to an artificial kidney machine about three times a week, or you may have dialysis done at home by a trained caregiver. Each session takes three to five hours. The second method may be done at home as well.

• Transplant. In some situations, the best option is a kidney transplant or a kidney-**pancreas** transplant. If you and your doctor decide on transplantation, you'll be evaluated to determine whether you're eligible for this surgery.

• Symptom management. If you choose not to have dialysis or a kidney transplant, your life expectancy generally would be only a few months. You may receive treatment to help keep you comfortable.

Potential future treatments

In the future, people with diabetic nephropathy may benefit from treatments being developed using regenerative medicine. These techniques may help reverse or slow kidney damage caused by the disease. For example, some researchers think that if a person's diabetes can be cured by a future treatment such as pancreas **islet** cell transplant or stem cell therapy, kidney function may improve. These therapies, however, are still investigational.

（1051 words）

◇ **Vocabulary**

diabetic nephropathy 糖尿病肾病

insulin ['ɪnsjəlɪn] *n.* [生化][药] 胰岛素

glomeruli [gləʊ'mer(j)ʊlaɪ] *n.* 小球，肾小球

nephrologist [ne'frʌlədʒɪst] *n.* 肾病学家

endocrinologist [ˌendəʊkrɪ'nɒlədʒɪst] *n.* 内分泌学家

microalbumin [maɪkrəʊlb'jʊmɪn] 微量白蛋白

inhibitor [ɪn'hɪbɪtə(r)] *n.* [助剂] 抑制剂，抗化剂；抑制者

mercury ['mɜːkjəri] *n.* 汞，水银，(温度计) 水银柱

hemoglobin [ˌhiːmə'gləʊbɪn] *n.* [生化] 血红蛋白(= haemoglobin)，血红素

phosphate ['fɒsfeɪt] *n.* 磷酸盐；皮膜化成

hemodialysis [hiːmədaɪ'ælɪsɪs] *n.* [临床] 血液透析，血液渗析

peritoneal [perɪtəʊ'niːəl] *adj.* 腹膜的

pancreas ['pæŋkriəs] *n.* [解剖] 胰腺

islet ['aɪlət] *n.* 小岛

Text D

Acute Kidney Failure

Acute kidney failure occurs when your kidneys suddenly become unable to filter waste products from your blood. When your kidneys lose their filtering ability, dangerous levels of wastes may accumulate, and your blood's chemical makeup may get out of balance. Acute kidney failure—also called acute renal failure or acute kidney injury—develops rapidly, usually in less than a few days. Acute kidney failure is most common in people who are already hospitalized, particularly in critically ill people who need intensive care. Acute kidney failure can be fatal and requires intensive treatment. However, acute kidney failure may be reversible. If you're otherwise in good health, you may recover normal or nearly normal kidney function.

Symptoms

Signs and symptoms of acute kidney failure may include:

- Decreased urine output, although occasionally urine output remains normal;
- Fluid retention, causing swelling in your legs, ankles or feet;
- Shortness of breath;
- Fatigue;
- Confusion;
- **Nausea**;
- Weakness;
- Irregular heartbeat;
- Chest pain or pressure;
- **Seizures** or **coma** in severe cases.

Sometimes acute kidney failure causes no signs or symptoms and is detected through lab tests done for another reason.

Causes

Acute kidney failure can occur when:

- You have a condition that slows blood flow to your kidneys;
- You experience direct damage to your kidneys;

- Your kidneys' urine drainage tubes (**ureters**) become blocked and wastes can't leave your body through your urine.

Impaired blood flow to the kidneys

Diseases and conditions that may slow blood flow to the kidneys and lead to kidney injury include:

- Blood or fluid loss;
- Blood pressure medications;
- Heart attack;
- Heart disease;
- Infection;
- Liver failure;
- Use of aspirin, ibuprofen (Advil, Motrin IB, others), naproxen sodium (Aleve, others) or related drugs;
- Severe allergic reaction (**anaphylaxis**);
- Severe burns;
- Severe dehydration.

Damage to the kidneys

These diseases, conditions and agents may damage the kidneys and lead to acute kidney failure:

- Blood clots in the veins and arteries in and around the kidneys;
- Cholesterol deposits that block blood flow in the kidneys;
- Glomerulonephritis, inflammation of the tiny filters in the kidneys (glomeruli);
- **Hemolytic uremic** syndrome, a condition that results from premature destruction of red blood cells;
- Infection, such as with the virus that causes coronavirus disease 2019 (COVID-19);
- Lupus, an immune system disorder causing glomerulonephritis;
- Medications, such as certain chemotherapy drugs, antibiotics and dyes used during imaging tests;
- **Scleroderma**, a group of rare diseases affecting the skin and connective tissues;
- **Thrombotic thrombocytopenic purpura**, a rare blood disorder;
- Toxins, such as alcohol, heavy metals and cocaine;
- Muscle tissue breakdown (**rhabdomyolysis**) that leads to kidney damage caused by toxins from muscle tissue destruction;
- Breakdown of tumor cells (**tumor lysis syndrome**), which leads to the release of toxins that can cause kidney injury.

Urine blockage in the kidneys

Diseases and conditions that block the passage of urine out of the body (urinary obstructions) and can lead to acute kidney injury include:

- Bladder cancer;
- Blood clots in the urinary tract;
- Cervical cancer;
- Colon cancer;
- Enlarged prostate;
- Kidney stones;
- Nerve damage involving the nerves that control the bladder;
- Prostate cancer.

Diagnosis

If your signs and symptoms suggest that you have acute kidney failure, your doctor may recommend certain tests and procedures to verify your diagnosis. These may include:

- Urine output measurements. Measuring how much you urinate in 24 hours may help your doctor determine the cause of your kidney failure.
- Urine tests. Analyzing a sample of your urine (urinalysis) may reveal abnormalities that suggest kidney failure.
- Blood tests. A sample of your blood may reveal rapidly rising levels of urea and creatinine—two substances used to measure kidney function.
- Imaging tests. Imaging tests such as ultrasound and computerized tomography may be used to help your doctor see your kidneys.
- Removing a sample of kidney tissue for testing. In some situations, your doctor may recommend a kidney biopsy to remove a small sample of kidney tissue for lab testing. Your doctor inserts a needle through your skin and into your kidney to remove the sample.

Treatment

Treatment for acute kidney failure typically requires a hospital stay. Most people with acute kidney failure are already hospitalized. How long you'll stay in the hospital depends on the reason for your acute kidney failure and how quickly your kidneys recover. In some cases, you may be able to recover at home.

Treating the underlying cause of your kidney injury

Treatment for acute kidney failure involves identifying the illness or injury that originally damaged your kidneys. Your treatment options depend on what's causing your kidney failure.

Treating complications until your kidneys recover

Your doctor will also work to prevent complications and allow your kidneys time to heal. Treatments that help prevent complications include:

• Treatments to balance the amount of fluids in your blood. If your acute kidney failure is caused by a lack of fluids in your blood, your doctor may recommend intravenous (IV) fluids. In other cases, acute kidney failure may cause you to have too much fluid, leading to swelling in your arms and legs. In these cases, your doctor may recommend medications (diuretics) to cause your body to expel extra fluids.

• Medications to control blood potassium. If your kidneys aren't properly filtering potassium from your blood, your doctor may prescribe calcium, glucose or sodium **polystyrene sulfonate** (Kionex) to prevent the accumulation of high levels of potassium in your blood. Too much potassium in the blood can cause dangerous irregular heartbeats (**arrhythmias**) and muscle weakness.

• Medications to restore blood calcium levels. If the levels of calcium in your blood drop too low, your doctor may recommend an infusion of calcium.

• Dialysis to remove toxins from your blood. If toxins build up in your blood, you may need temporary hemodialysis—often referred to simply as dialysis—to help remove toxins and excess fluids from your body while your kidneys heal. Dialysis may also help remove excess potassium from your body. During dialysis, a machine pumps blood out of your body through an artificial kidney (dialyzer) that filters out waste. The blood is then returned to your body.

(1046 words)

◆ **Vocabulary**

acute kidney failure 急性肾衰竭
nausea ['nɔːziə] *n.* 恶心，晕船
seizure ['siːʒə(r)] *n.*（疾病的）突然发作，痛性发作；夺取，捕获

coma ['kəʊmə] *n.* [医] 昏迷
ureter [jʊ'riːtə] *n.* 尿管；[解剖] 输尿管
anaphylaxis [ˌænəfɪ'læksɪs] *n.* [医] 过敏性，过敏性反应

hemolytic [hiːˈmɒlɪtɪk] *adj.* [生理][免疫] 溶血的

uremic [jʊˈriːmɪk] *adj.* [泌尿] 尿毒症的

scleroderma [sklɪərəˈdɜːmə] *n.* [内科] 硬皮病

thrombotic [θrɑːmˈbɒtɪk] *adj.* 血栓形成的

thrombocytopenic [ˈθrɒmbəʊˌsaɪtəˈpiːnɪk] *adj.* 血小板减少的

purpura [ˈpɜːpjʊrə] *n.* [内科] 紫癜

rhabdomyolysis [ræbdəʊmaɪˈəʊlɪsɪs] *n.* 横纹肌溶解

tumor lysis syndrome 肿瘤溶解综合征

polystyrene [ˌpɒliˈstaɪriːn] *n.* [高分子] 聚苯乙烯

sulfonate [ˈsʌlfəneɪt] *n.* 磺化，磺酸盐（= sulphonate）*v.* 使……磺化

arrhythmia [əˈrɪðmɪə] *n.* 心律不齐，[内科] 心律失常

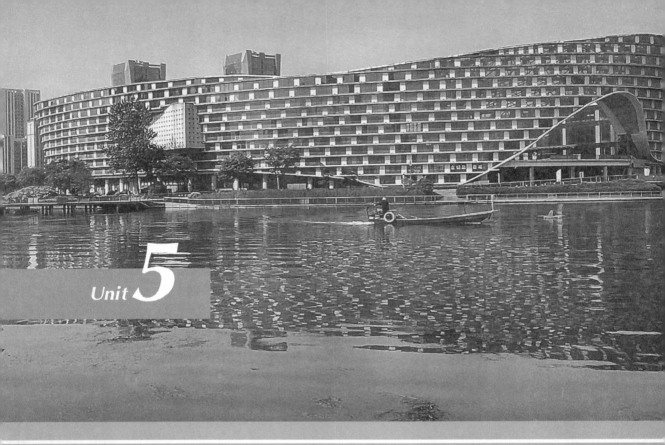

Some Common Diseases of the Reproductive System

✓参考答案
✓微课等资源

Text A

Cervicitis

Cervicitis is an inflammation of the **cervix**. The cervix is a narrow passage that connects the uterus and **vagina**. Every month, **menstrual** blood comes out of the uterus through the cervix and into the vagina. When a woman has a baby, the cervix expands to allow the baby to move into the birth canal. If something irritates the cervix and it becomes inflamed, the condition is called cervicitis.

Symptoms

Symptoms of cervicitis may include:

- Vaginal itching or irritation;
- Bleeding between periods;
- Pain when having sex;
- Bleeding after sex;
- Pain during a cervical exam;
- Frequent and painful urination;
- Unusual gray or white discharge that may smell;
- A pressurized feeling in the **pelvis**;
- Lowerback pain;
- Abdominal pain.

Some women may not experience any symptoms when they have cervicitis. Severe cervicitis may lead to a thick, yellow or green vaginal discharge that resembles pus.

Causes

Cases of cervicitis may be mild or severe. Cervicitis is often caused by a sexually transmitted infection (STI), such as:

- Chlamydia;
- Gonorrhea;
- **Trichomoniasis**;
- Genital **herpes**;
- Mycoplasma;

- **Ureaplasma**.

Other causes of cervicitis include:

- Allergies: If someone is allergic to spermicides, **douches**, or **latex** in condoms, these may cause the cervix to become inflamed.
- Irritation: Inserting tampons, **pessaries**, or diaphragms may irritate or injure the cervix. Cervicitis may also develop if these items are left in place longer than directed.
- Bacterial imbalance: If harmful bacteria overwhelm the healthful bacteria in the vagina, this may cause bacterial **vaginosis**. An inflamed cervix may be a symptom of this.
- Pregnancy: This can affect hormone levels and lead to cervicitis as the cervix is much more sensitive at this time.
- Cancer or cancer treatment: Treatment for cancer or advanced stages of cervical cancer itself may affect cervical tissue. This is rare but may lead to symptoms of cervicitis.

Cervicitis may be either acute or chronic. Acute cervicitis is typically caused by an infection and is best treated medically. Chronic cervicitis is not typically caused by an infection. Symptoms may be milder but last longer. Some people may want to treat chronic cervicitis at home, using natural remedies that will complement medical treatments. However, it is essential to discuss this strategy with a healthcare provider to ensure the person receive the correct treatment.

Diagnosis

If a woman thinks that she may have cervicitis, it is a good idea to see a doctor to get a full diagnosis. The doctor will carry out a **pelvic** exam to examine the cervix and may take a **swab**. This helps the doctor to collect cells and fluids. These may be tested for abnormalities or examined under a microscope.

To reach a full diagnosis, the doctor may also test for STIs. Treating these may heal the inflammation.

Risk factors

You're at greater risk of cervicitis if you:

- Engage in high-risk sexual behavior, such as unprotected sex, sex with multiple partners or sex with someone who engages in high-risk behaviors.
- Began having sexual intercourse at an early age.

- Have a history of sexually transmitted infections.

Prevention

To reduce your risk of cervicitis from sexually transmitted infections, use condoms consistently and correctly each time you have sex. Condoms are very effective against the spread of STIs, such as gonorrhea and chlamydia, which can lead to cervicitis. Being in a long-term relationship in which both you and your uninfected partner are committed to having sex with each other exclusively can lower your odds of an STI.

Complications

If left untreated, cervicitis may lead to complications. These may include:

- Pelvic inflammatory disease;
- Infertility;
- **Ectopic** pregnancy, where a fertilized egg implants outside of the **womb**;
- Chronic pelvic pain.

Treatment

Doctors commonly prescribe antibiotics as a treatment for cervicitis. These drugs help to clear the infection, which helps to treat symptoms. If cervicitis is caused by an STI, the doctor can advise on the best course of treatments. STIs are often treatable with antibiotics. If a foreign body is irritating the cervix, a doctor will remove the object and may prescribe antibiotics.

Natural treatment options

Acute cervicitis that is caused by an infection is best treated medically, as it is essential to clear up the infection. If a woman has chronic cervicitis with mild symptoms, she may choose to use home remedies to help ease the symptoms. A person should always use home remedies alongside medical treatments. They are not intended to replace them. Home remedies that may help treat cervicitis include:

- Traditional Chinese medicine: A 2014 study found that traditional Chinese medicinal treatments, including specific Chinese herbs, may be effective in the treatment of cervicitis. The herbs were reported to have an anti-inflammatory effect.

• Eating yogurt or taking **probiotic** supplements: Yogurt contains healthful bacteria called probiotics. Probiotics are also available in supplement form and are available to buy online. A 2014 study suggests that probiotics may help treat bacterial vaginosis, which is one cause of cervicitis.

• Eating garlic or taking a garlic supplement: Garlic has strong antibacterial properties. Another 2014 study found that taking garlic supplements may also help treat bacterial vaginosis.

It is a good idea to seek a diagnosis and advice from a doctor before deciding on a course of treatment. These alternative treatments need further studies as they are not considered first-line treatment for cervicitis or vaginal infections at this time.

Home remedies that support vaginal and cervical health and may prevent cervicitis include:

• Drinking green tea: A 2014 study suggested green tea may have a protective role in reducing the risk of **ovarian** and **endometrial** cancers.

• Avoiding irritants: Avoiding douches, tampons, diaphragms, and scented soaps reduces the risk of irritation.

• Wearing loose cotton underwear: Breathable underwear reduces the buildup of moisture and bacteria that can lead to infection.

• Using condoms during sex: This reduces the risk of STIs, one of the leading causes of cervicitis.

Outlook

Cervicitis is typically treatable. Home treatments and prevention strategies should be used alongside, not instead of medical treatment. Acute cervicitis caused by infections is best treated medically to avoid complications. If someone thinks they may have cervicitis, they should speak to their doctor.

（1034 words）

◆ **Vocabulary**

cervicitis [sɜːvɪˈsaɪtɪs] n. ［妇产］子宫颈炎
cervix [ˈsɜːvɪks] n. 子宫颈, 颈部
vagina [vəˈdʒaɪnə] n. ［解剖］阴道
menstrual [ˈmenstruəl] adj. 月经的, 每月的

pelvis [ˈpelvɪs] n. 骨盆（复数 pelvises 或 pelves）
trichomoniasis [ˌtrɪkəʊməˈnaɪəsɪs] n. 滴虫病, 阴道滴虫病

herpes ['hɜːpiːz] n. [皮肤] 疱疹

ureaplasma [juəriːp'læzmə] n. 尿素原体，脲原体

douche ['duːʃ] n.（避孕用）阴道冲洗器

latex ['leɪteks] n. 乳胶，乳液

pessary ['pesəri] n. 子宫帽，子宫托；阴道栓

vaginosis [vædʒɪ'nəʊsɪs] [医] 阴道病（炎）

pelvic ['pelvɪk] adj. 骨盆的

swab [swɒb] n. [外科] 拭子；医用棉签

vt. 打扫，擦拭；涂抹（药）于

ectopic [ek'tɒpɪk] adj. 异位的，异常的

womb [wuːm] n. [解剖] 子宫；发源地

probiotic [ˌprəʊbaɪ'ɒtɪk] adj. 益菌的
n. 益生微生物，益生菌

ovarian [əʊ'veərɪən] adj. [解剖] 卵巢的，子房的

endometrial [ˌendəʊ'miːtrɪəl] adj. [解剖] 子宫内膜的

◈ Exercises

Ⅰ. **Decide whether the following sentences are *True* or *False* according to the text.**

1. When a woman has a baby, the cervix shrinks to allow the baby to move into the birth canal.

2. Severe cervicitis may lead to a thick, yellow or green vaginal discharge that resembles mucus.

3. Cervicitis is often caused by a STI, such as chlamydia, gonorrhea, trichomoniasis, etc.

4. Pregnancy is a cause of cervitis, but bacterial imbalance is not a cause of it.

5. Chronic cervicitis may be milder but last longer. Some patients may treat chronic cervicitis at home with the guidance from a healthcare provider.

6. Generally speaking, doctors commonly prescribe antibiotics to treat cervicitis, but STIs can not be treated with antibiotics.

7. Because traditional Chinese medicine has an anti-inflammatory effect, it may be effective to treat cervicitis.

8. Although garlic has strong antibacterial properties, it may not help treat bacterial vaginosis.

9. Drinking green tea is a way that may prevent cervicitis and eating yogurt may help treat cervicitis.

10. Cervicitis may lead to infertility, but not chronic pelvic pain.

Ⅱ. **Fill in the blanks with the proper form of words in the box.**

cervicitis	vagina	menstrual	gonorrhea	ovarian
womb	vaginosis	endometrial	pelvis	herpes

1. _____ is a kind of inflammatory skin disease caused by a herpes virus

and characterized by formation of small vesicles in clusters.

2. _____ is a major female hormone-responsive secondary sex organ of the reproductive system in humans and most other mammals.

3. _____ is common infectious disease caused by a bacterium, involving chiefly the mucous membranes of the genitourinary tract.

4. _____ cancer is a cancer that arises from the endometrium (the lining of the uterus or womb).

5. _____ cancer is cancer of the ovaries, the egg-releasing and hormone-producing organs of the female reproductive tract.

6. Bacterial _____ is a disease of the vagina caused by excessive growth of bacteria.

7. The _____ is either the lower part of the trunk of the human body between the abdomen and the thighs or the skeleton embedded in it.

8. In mammals, the _____ is the elastic, muscular part of the female genital tract.

9. The average length of a woman's _____ cycle is 28 days.

10. _____ is inflammation of the uterine cervix.

Ⅲ. Translation: translate the passage into Chinese.

Polycystic ovary syndrome (PCOS) is a hormonal disorder common among women of reproductive age. Women with PCOS may have infrequent or prolonged menstrual periods or excess male hormone (androgen) levels. The ovaries may develop numerous small collections of fluid (follicles) and fail to regularly release eggs. The exact cause of PCOS is unknown. Early diagnosis and treatment along with weight loss may reduce the risk of long-term complications such as type 2 diabetes and heart disease.

Signs and symptoms of PCOS often develop around the time of the first menstrual period during puberty. Sometimes PCOS develops later, for example, in response to substantial weight gain. Signs and symptoms of PCOS vary. A diagnosis of PCOS is made when you experience at least two of these signs:

• Irregular periods. Infrequent, irregular or prolonged menstrual cycles are the most common sign of PCOS. For example, you might have fewer than nine periods a year, more than 35 days between periods and abnormally heavy periods.

• Excess androgen. Elevated levels of male hormones may result in physical signs, such as excess facial and body hair (hirsutism), and occasionally severe acne and male-pattern baldness.

- Polycystic ovaries. Your ovaries might be enlarged and contain follicles that surround the eggs. As a result, the ovaries might fail to function regularly. PCOS signs and symptoms are typically more severe if you're obese.

The exact cause of PCOS isn't known. Factors that might play a role include:

- Excess insulin. Insulin is the hormone produced in the pancreas that allows cells to use sugar, your body's primary energy supply. If your cells become resistant to the action of insulin, then your blood sugar levels can rise and your body might produce more insulin. Excess insulin might increase androgen production, causing difficulty with ovulation.
- Low-grade inflammation. This term is used to describe white blood cells' production of substances to fight infection. Research has shown that women with PCOS have a type of low-grade inflammation that stimulates polycystic ovaries to produce androgens, which can lead to heart and blood vessel problems.
- Heredity. Research suggests that certain genes might be linked to PCOS.
- Excess androgen. The ovaries produce abnormally high levels of androgen, resulting in hirsutism and acne.

(372 words)

Ⅳ. Give a presentation.

Dictate the causes, symptoms, treatments, etc. of Cervicitis in English with 3—4 students. Try to use the formal expression, especially related medical terminology when you make your presentation.

Ⅴ. Write a certificate for an on-campus student.

根据下列内容写一份在读证明：

李丽(学号 123456)，2018 年被天津医科大学临床医学院临床医学专业录取，现为校临床医学专业四年级本科生，拟毕业时间 2023 年 7 月。天津医科大学 2022 年 1 月 18 日。

Text B

Prostatitis

The prostate is a walnut-sized gland that all men have. It's found below the bladder and in front of the **rectum**. The job of the prostate is to make fluid that contains **sperm** (**semen**). This fluid protects the sperm when they travel toward a female's egg.

Prostatitis is a common condition that may be caused by infection or inflammation of the prostate and sometimes the area around it. It is seen most commonly in men under 50 years and some studies suggest that up to 10% of men suffer from prostatitis. There are several types of prostatitis, each with a range of symptoms. Some men with prostatitis have a great deal of discomfort and pain, which may be in the pelvic area, **testicles**, or lower back. They may have pain when they urinate or **ejaculate**. Other patients may have symptoms similar to patients with **BPH**. Other patients are not really bothered by their symptoms.

Causes

Although the causes of prostatitis are not clearly known, there are many theories about why you may contract it. Prostatitis from bacteria may be a result of a backward flow of urine into the prostate. This infected urine may be a result of a recent bladder infection, an abnormality of your urinary tract, a result of a catheterization or recent surgery. Non bacterial prostatitis may be caused by other organisms, or clogging of the prostate ducts. Another theory of the cause of non bacterial prostatitis is that the nerves and muscles around the prostate are not working correctly, and may be causing too much tension at the outflow of the bladder and at the level of the **pelvic floor**. Also, the nerves in the area of the prostate may have become oversensitive over time, thus causing discomfort and pain in that area. As a result of the causes of non bacterial prostatitis being less well understood, and the symptoms of all the types of prostatitis being very similar, diagnosis and treatment can be a frustrating experience for both the patient and the doctor.

Symptoms

There are four types of prostatitis. Each has its own set of symptoms and causes. These include:

Acute bacterial prostatitis. Your urinary tract is made up of your kidneys, bladder, and the tubes that pass between them. If bacteria from here finds its way into your prostate, you can get an infection. This type of prostatitis comes on quickly. You might suddenly have:

- Urgent need to **pee** but only a little comes out, or you have to get to the toilet quickly to prevent an accident;
  - High fever;
  - Chills;
  - Trouble peeing;
  - Pain around the base of your **penis** or behind your **scrotum**;
  - **Cloudy urine**.

Acute bacterial prostatitis is a severe condition. If you notice these symptoms, seek medical care right away.

Chronic bacterial prostatitis. This is more common in older men. It's a milder bacterial infection that can linger for several months. Some men get it after they've had a urinary tract infection (UTI) or acute bacterial prostatitis. The symptoms of chronic bacterial prostatitis often come and go. This makes them easy to miss. With this condition, you might sometimes have:

- An urgent need to pee, often in the middle of the night;
- Painful urination;
- Pain after you ejaculate (release semen at **orgasm**);
- Lower back pain;
- Rectum pain;
- A "heavy" feeling behind your scrotum;
- Blood in your semen;
- Urinary blockage (difficulty peeing or a weak urine stream).

*Chronic prostatitis/**chronic pelvic pain syndrome** (CP/CPPS).* This is the most common type of prostatitis. It shares many of the same signs as bacterial prostatitis. The difference is that when tests are run, no bacteria are present with this type. Doctors aren't sure what causes CP/CPPS. Triggers include stress, nearby nerve damage, and physical injury. Chemicals in your urine or a UTI you had in the past may play a role. The main symptom of CP/CPPS is pain that lasts more than 3 months in at least one of these body parts:

- Penis (often at the tip)
- Scrotum

- Between your scrotum and rectum (the perineum)
- Lower abdomen

You may also have pain when you pee or ejaculate. You might not be able to hold your urine, or you may have to pee more than 8 times a day. A weak urine stream is another common symptom of CP/CPPS.

Asymptomatic prostatitis. Men who have this type of prostatitis have an inflamed prostate but no symptoms. You may only learn you have it if your doctor does a blood test that checks your prostate health. Asymptomatic prostatitis doesn't need any treatment, but it can lead to infertility.

Diagnosis

Your **urologist** will ask you questions about the symptoms you have and are currently experiencing and about your medical history. You may be asked to complete a chronic prostatitis symptom questionnaire.

You will then be examined, and this will include an examination of your **tummy** (abdomen), testicles and a digital rectal examination (DRE) to feel the prostate gland. A urine dipstick will be performed to see if there is any evidence of blood in the urine or of a urinary infection, and the specimen may then be sent off for a urine culture.

Your PSA (prostate specific antigen) blood test may be taken, although the value of this is uncertain. Your urologist may ask you to perform a flow test to see how fast you pass urine. You will need to have a comfortably full bladder to do this. It involves passing urine as usual, but into a **funneled tube** which collects the urine and can measure how much you pass per second. Following this you will have a bladder scan, which takes just a minute and involves passing an ultrasound probe over the lower part of your tummy to see how much urine you leave in your bladder.

You may also need to undergo a cystoscopy to examine the prostate and bladder further. This test is completed in the hospital, and takes about ten minutes. A small telescope is inserted into the urethra after an **anaesthetic gel** is applied. This telescope allows the specialist to see your prostate and bladder, and see if there are any abnormalities or inflammation.

Treatment

Treatment of prostatitis depends very much on the cause. The three main types of prostatitis are acute bacterial, chronic bacterial, and chronic pelvic pain syndrome. These are described in more detail below.

Acute bacterial prostatitis. If you are very symptomatic, or sick, you may need to be admitted to the hospital to be treated with **intravenous** antibiotics. If your symptoms are not severe, antibiotics taken in a pill form can be effective. The antibiotics may be prescribed for up to a month, and it is very important that you take the entire course prescribed.

Chronic bacterial prostatitis. This is also treated by antibiotics, but they are required for one to three months. Again, it is very important that you take the pills for the length of time prescribed by the doctor.

Chronic pelvic pain syndrome. As this form is not caused by bacteria, antibiotics will not help. Your doctor may try antibiotics, initially, however. Treatment of this condition is difficult, and many patients learn how to manage their symptoms.

Treatment options include tablets that relax the tissue of the prostate called alpha blockers.

A number of other treatments may be tried, and these include:

- Anti-inflammatory pain killers (eg: ibuprofen or **diclofenac**);
- **Tricyclic** antidepressant tablets (eg: amitryptilline);
- Prostatic massage, to help remove prostatic secretions;
- **Physiotherapy**, to help learn to relax the pelvic floor.

More natural methods to help symptoms might include:

- Warm baths;
- Diet changes (avoid caffeine, alcohol, spicy or acidic foods);
- Relaxation exercises;
- Frequent ejaculation.

(1307 words)

Vocabulary

rectum ['rektəm] n. 直肠 [复数 rectums 或 recta]
sperm [spɜːm] n. 精子,精液
semen ['siːmən] n. 精液,精子
testicle [testɪkəl] n. [解剖] 睾丸
ejaculate [ɪ'dʒækjʊleɪt] vt. 突然说出,射出 vi. 射精,射出液体

BPH (benign prostatic hyperplasia) 良性前列腺增生
pelvic floor [ˌpelvɪk 'flɔː(r)] [解剖] 骨盆底
pee [piː] v. 撒尿,小便　n. 撒尿,尿
penis ['piːnɪs] n. [解剖] 阴茎,阳物
scrotum ['skrəʊtəm] n. [解剖] 阴囊

cloudy urine [ˈklaʊdi ˈjʊrɪn] 混浊尿

orgasm [ˈɔːgæzəm] n. [生理] 性高潮,极度兴奋

chronic pelvic pain syndrome 慢性盆腔疼痛综合征

asymptomatic [æˌsɪmptəˈmætɪk] adj. 无症状的

urologist [jʊəˈrɒlədʒɪst] n. 泌尿科医师

tummy [ˈtʌmi] n. 肚子,胃

funneled tube 漏斗管,长梗漏斗

anaesthetic gel 麻醉凝胶

intravenous [ˌɪntrəˈviːnəs] adj. 静脉内的

diclofenac [dɪklɒfeˈnæk] n. 双氯芬酸

tricyclic [traɪˈsaɪklɪk] adj. 三环的

physiotherapy [ˌfɪziəʊˈθerəpi] n. 物理疗法

◆ **Exercises**

Ⅰ. **Decide whether the following sentences are *True* or *False* according to the text.**

1. The prostate is below your bladder and behind your rectum. Its function is to make fluid that contains semen.

2. Prostatitis may be caused by infection or inflammation of the prostate and sometimes the area around it.

3. Some studies show that up to 10% of men suffer from prostatitis, most commonly in men under 50 years.

4. If bacteria finds its way into your prostate from urinary tract, you can get an infection, resulting in chronic bacterial prostatitis.

5. Chronic bacterial prostatitis is more common in older men and can linger for several months.

6. There are four types of prostatitis, but each type has the common symptoms and causes.

7. CPPS shares many of the same signs as bacterial prostatitis. When tests are done, bacteria are still present with this type.

8. As a patient of acute bacterial prostatitis, if you feel better, you can stop taking the medication and your infection will not return.

9. Anti-inflammatory pain killers as well as relaxation exercises can treat chronic pelvic pain syndrome.

10. People with chronic bacterial prostatitis should take the pills for the length of time prescribed by the doctor.

II. Fill in the blanks with the proper form of words in the box.

cystoscopy	prostatitis	testicles	scrotum	sperm
rectum	analgesics	biopsy	urologist	ejaculate

1. The _____ is the final straight portion of the large intestine in humans and some other mammals.

2. A man's _____ are the two reproductive glands that produce sperm and are contained in the scrotum.

3. _____ is a diagnostic procedure that is used to look at the bladder, collect urine samples, and examine the prostate gland.

4. _____ are those drugs that mainly provide pain relief.

5. _____ refers to examination of cells or tissues removed from a living organism.

6. _____ is a physician specialised in diagnosing and treating diseases of the genitourinary tract.

7. Each male _____ will contain up to 300 million sperm.

8. A man's _____ is the bag of skin that contains his testicles.

9. _____ is inflammation of the prostate gland.

10. Conception occurs when a single _____ fuses with an egg.

III. Translation: translate the passage into Chinese.

Orchitis is inflammation of one or both of a man's testicles, usually because of an infection. Orchitis can result from the spread of bacteria through your blood from somewhere else in your body. It also can be a progression of epididymitis, an infection of the tube that carries semen out of your testicles. This is called epididymo-orchitis.

Most cases of orchitis are acute, which means you have sudden, severe pain in one or both testicles that may spread to your groin (the area where your upper thigh meets your lower belly). You also may have: testicles that appear tender, swollen, and red or purple, a heavy feeling in the swollen testicle, blood in your semen, high fever, nausea, vomiting, pain with urination, pain from straining with a bowel movement, pain with intercourse, feeling ill. Orchitis causes an area of pain and swelling in the testicle for one to several days. Later, the infection spreads to involving the whole testicle.

Most cases of orchitis—and epididymo-orchitis—need antibiotics to cure the infection and prevent its spread. Most men can be treated with antibiotics at home for at least 10 days. If your prostate is involved, you'll probably need a longer course of medication. If you have a high fever, nausea, or vomiting, or if you're very ill, you may need to be admitted to a hospital to get antibiotics directly into a vein (IV). Mumps orchitis will clear up over 1 to 3 weeks. Just treat your symptoms with home care. Young sexually active men should make sure all of their sexual partners are treated. Avoid sex or use condoms until all partners have finished their full course of antibiotics and are symptom-free.

(290 words)

IV. Give a presentation.

Dictate the causes, symptoms, treatments, etc. of Prostatitis in English with 3—4 students. Try to use the formal expression, especially related medical terminology when you make your presentation.

V. Write a working certificate.

根据下列内容,写一份在职证明。

张翔,男,身份证号码:123456789123654132,自 2011 年 7 月 8 日至今为我院泌尿外科医生。上海人民医院人事部主任王力,2021 年 8 月 20 日。

Text C

Vaginitis

Vaginitis is an inflammation of the vagina that can result in discharge, itching and pain. The cause is usually a change in the balance of vaginal bacteria or an infection. Reduced estrogen levels after menopause and some skin disorders also can cause vaginitis.

The most common types of vaginitis are:

• Bacterial vaginosis. This results from an overgrowth of the bacteria naturally found in your vagina, which upsets the natural balance.

• **Yeast infections**. These are usually caused by a naturally occurring fungus called Candida **albicans**.

• Trichomoniasis. This is caused by a parasite and is often sexually transmitted.

Treatment depends on the type of vaginitis you have.

Symptoms

Vaginitis signs and symptoms can include:

• Change in color, odor or amount of discharge from your vagina;
• Vaginal itching or irritation;
• Pain during sex;
• Painful urination;
• Light vaginal bleeding or spotting.

If you have vaginal discharge, the characteristics of the discharge might indicate the type of vaginitis you have. Examples include:

• Bacterial vaginosis. You might develop a grayish-white, **foul**-smelling discharge. The odor, often described as a fishy odor, might be more obvious after sex.

• Yeast infection. The main symptom is itching, but you might have a thick white discharge that resembles cottage cheese.

• Trichomoniasis. An infection called trichomoniasis can cause a greenish-yellow, sometimes **frothy** discharge.

Causes

The causes depend on what type of vaginitis you have:

• Bacterial vaginosis. This most common type of vaginitis results from a change of the bacteria found in your vagina, upsetting the balance. What causes the imbalance is unknown. It's possible to have bacterial vaginosis without symptoms.

This type of vaginitis seems to be linked to but not caused by sex—especially if you have multiple sex partners or a new sex partner—but it also occurs in women who aren't sexually active.

• Yeast infections. These occur when there's an overgrowth of a fungal organism—usually Candida albicans—in your vagina. C. albicans also causes infections in other moist areas of your body, such as in your mouth, skin folds and **nail beds**. The fungus can also cause **diaper rash**.

• Trichomoniasis. This common sexually transmitted infection is caused by a microscopic, one-celled parasite called Trichomonas vaginalis. This organism spreads during sex with someone who has the infection.

In men, the organism usually infects the urinary tract, but often it causes no symptoms. In women, trichomoniasis typically infects the vagina, and might cause symptoms. It also increases women's risk of getting other sexually transmitted infections.

• Noninfectious vaginitis. Vaginal sprays, douches, perfumed soaps, scented detergents and **spermicidal** products can cause an allergic reaction or irritate **vulvar** and vaginal tissues. Foreign objects, such as toilet paper or forgotten tampons, in the vagina also can irritate vaginal tissues.

• Genitourinary syndrome of menopause (vaginal **atrophy**). Reduced estrogen levels after menopause or surgical removal of your ovaries can cause the vaginal lining to thin, sometimes resulting in vaginal irritation, burning and dryness.

Prevention

Good hygiene might prevent some types of vaginitis from recurring and relieve some symptoms:

• Avoid baths, hot tubs and **whirlpool** spas.
• Avoid irritants. These include scented tampons, pads, douches and scented soaps. **Rinse** soap from your outer genital area after a shower and dry the area well to prevent irritation. Don't use harsh soaps, such as those with

deodorant or antibacterial action, or bubble bath.

• Wipe from front to back after using the toilet. Doing so avoids spreading **fecal** bacteria to your vagina.

Other things that might help prevent vaginitis include:

• Avoid douching. Your vagina doesn't require cleansing other than regular showering. Repetitive douching disrupts the good organisms that live in the vagina and can increase your risk of vaginal infection. Douching won't clear up a vaginal infection.

• Practice safer sex. Using a condom and limiting the number of sex partners can help.

• Wear cotton underwear. Also wear **pantyhose** with a cotton crotch. Consider not wearing underwear to bed. Yeast thrives in moist environments.

Diagnosis

To diagnose vaginitis, your health care provider is likely to:

• Review your medical history. This includes your history of vaginal or sexually transmitted infections.

• Perform a pelvic exam. During the pelvic exam, your health care provider might use an instrument (**speculum**) to look inside your vagina for inflammation and discharge.

• Collect a sample for lab testing. Your health care provider might collect a sample of cervical or vaginal discharge for lab testing to confirm what kind of vaginitis you have.

• Perform pH testing. Your health care provider might test your vaginal pH by applying a pH test stick or pH paper to the wall of your vagina. An elevated pH can indicate either bacteria vaginosis or trichomoniasis. However, pH testing alone is not a reliable diagnostic test.

Treatment

A variety of organisms and conditions can cause vaginitis, so treatment targets the specific cause:

• Bacterial vaginosis. For this type of vaginitis, your health care provider might prescribe **metronidazole** tablets (Flagyl) that you take by mouth or metronidazole gel (MetroGel) that you apply to the affected area. Other treatments include **clindamycin** (Cleocin) cream that you apply to your vagina, clindamycin tablets you take by mouth or capsules you put in your vagina. **Tinidazole** (Tindamax) or **secnidazole** (Solosec) are taken by mouth.

Bacterial vaginosis can recur after treatment.

- Yeast infections. Yeast infections usually are treated with an over-the-counter antifungal cream or **suppository**. Yeast infections might also be treated with a prescription oral antifungal medication, such as **fluconazole** (Diflucan).

The advantages of over-the-counter treatment are convenience, cost and not waiting to see your health care provider. However, you might have something other than a yeast infection. Using the wrong medicine might delay an accurate diagnosis and proper treatment.

- Trichomoniasis. Your health care provider may prescribe metronidazole (Flagyl) or tinidazole (Tindamax) tablets.

- Genitourinary syndrome of menopause (vaginal atrophy). Estrogen—in the form of vaginal creams, tablets or rings—can treat this condition. This treatment is available by prescription from your health care provider, after other risk factors and possible complications are reviewed.

- Noninfectious vaginitis. To treat this type of vaginitis, you need to pinpoint the source of the irritation and avoid it. Possible sources include new soap, laundry detergent, sanitary napkins or tampons.

（1047 words）

◆ Vocabulary

vaginitis [ˌvædʒəˈnaɪtɪs] n. [医]阴道炎

yeast infection 酵母菌感染

albicans [ˈælbɪkəns] n. 白体，乳头状体
    adj. 白色的

foul [faʊl] adj. 恶臭的，邪恶的，污秽的

frothy [ˈfrɒθi] adj. 起泡的，多泡的，空洞的

nail bed 甲床

diaper rash 尿布疹

spermicidal [ˌspɜːmɪˈsaɪdl] adj. 杀精子的

vulvar [ˈvʌlvə] adj. 外阴的，会阴部的

atrophy [ˈætrəfi] n. 萎缩，萎缩症

whirlpool [ˈwɜːlˌpuːl] n. 漩涡

rinse [rɪns] v. 清洗，冲洗

fecal [ˈfiːkl] adj. 排泄物的

pantyhose [ˈpæntiˌhəʊz] n. 连裤袜

speculum [ˈspekjələm] n. 反射镜，[医]窥器

metronidazole [metrəˈnaɪdəzəʊl] n. [药]灭滴灵，甲硝哒唑(抗滴虫药)

clindamycin [klɪndəˈmaɪsɪn] n. [药]克林霉素

tinidazole [tɪnɪdˈəəʊl] n. [药]磺甲硝咪唑

secnidazole [seknɪdˈəəʊl] n. [药]塞克硝唑

suppository [səˈpɒzətri] n. 栓剂，塞剂，坐药

fluconazole [fluːˈkɒnəzəʊl] n. [药]氟康唑，抗真菌药

Text D

Genital Warts

Genital **warts** are one of the most common types of sexually transmitted infections. Nearly all sexually active people will become infected with at least one type of human **papilloma** virus (HPV), the virus that causes genital warts, at some point during their lives. Genital warts affect the moist tissues of the genital area. They can look like small, flesh-colored bumps or have a cauliflower-like appearance. In many cases, the warts are too small to be visible. Some strains of genital HPV can cause genital warts, while others can cause cancer. Vaccines can help protect against certain strains of genital HPV.

Symptoms

In women, genital warts can grow on the vulva, the walls of the vagina, the area between the external genitals and the anus, the anal canal, and the cervix. In men, they may occur on the tip or shaft of the penis, the scrotum, or the anus. Genital warts can also develop in the mouth or throat of a person. The signs and symptoms of genital warts include:

- Small, flesh-colored, brown or pink swellings in your genital area;
- A cauliflower-like shape caused by several warts close together;
- Itching or discomfort in your genital area;
- Bleeding with intercourse.

Genital warts can be so small and flat as to be invisible. Rarely, however, genital warts can multiply into large clusters, in someone with a suppressed immune system.

Causes

The human papilloma virus (HPV) causes warts. There are more than 40 strains of HPV that affect the genital area. Genital warts are almost always spread through sexual contact. Your warts don't have to be visible for you to spread the infection to your sexual partner.

Complications

HPV infection complications can include:

• Cancer. Cervical cancer has been closely linked with genital HPV infection. Certain types of HPV also are associated with cancers of the vulva, anus, penis, and mouth and throat. HPV infection doesn't always lead to cancer, but it's important for women to have regular Pap tests, particularly those who've been infected with higher risk types of HPV.

• Problems during pregnancy. Rarely during pregnancy, warts can enlarge, making it difficult to urinate. Warts on the vaginal wall can inhibit the stretching of vaginal tissues during childbirth. Large warts on the vulva or in the vagina can bleed when stretched during delivery. Extremely rarely, a baby born to a mother with genital warts develops warts in the throat. The baby might need surgery to keep the airway from being blocked.

Diagnosis

Genital warts are often diagnosed by appearance. Sometimes a biopsy might be necessary.

Pap tests

For women, it's important to have regular pelvic exams and Pap tests, which can help detect vaginal and cervical changes caused by genital warts or the early signs of cervical cancer. During a Pap test, your doctor uses a device called a speculum to hold open your vagina and see the passage between your vagina and your uterus (cervix). He or she will then use a long-handled tool to collect a small sample of cells from the cervix. The cells are examined with a microscope for abnormalities.

HPV test

Only a few types of genital HPV have been linked to cervical cancer. A sample of cervical cells, taken during a Pap test, can be tested for these cancer-causing HPV strains. This test is generally reserved for women ages 30 and older. It isn't as useful for younger women because for them, HPV usually goes away without treatment.

Treatment

If your warts aren't causing discomfort, you might not need treatment. But if you have itching, burning and pain, or if you're concerned about spreading the infection, your doctor can help you clear an outbreak with medications or surgery. However, warts often return after treatment. There is no treatment for the virus itself.

Medications

Genital wart treatments that can be applied directly to your skin include:

- **Imiquimod** (Aldara, Zyclara). This cream appears to boost your immune system's ability to fight genital warts. Avoid sexual contact while the cream is on your skin. It might weaken condoms and diaphragms and irritate your partner's skin. One possible side effect is skin redness. Other side effects might include blisters, body aches or pain, rashes, and fatigue.
- **Podophyllin** and **podofilox** (Condylox). Podophyllin is a plant-based resin that destroys genital wart tissue. Your doctor applies this solution. Podofilox contains the same active compound, but you can apply it at home. Never apply podofilox internally. Additionally, this medication isn't recommended for use during pregnancy. Side effects can include mild skin irritation, sores or pain.
- **Trichloroacetic** acid. This chemical treatment burns off genital warts, and can be used for internal warts. Side effects can include mild skin irritation, sores or pain.
- Sinecatechins (Veregen). This cream is used for treatment of external genital warts and warts in or around the anal canal. Side effects, such as reddening of the skin, itching or burning, and pain, are often mild.

Don't try to treat genital warts with over-the-counter wart removers. These medications aren't intended for use in the genital area.

Surgery

You might need surgery to remove larger warts, warts that don't respond to medications or, if you're pregnant, warts that your baby can be exposed to during delivery. Surgical options include:

- Freezing with liquid nitrogen (**cryotherapy**). Freezing works by causing a blister to form around your wart. As your skin heals, the lesions slough off, allowing new skin to appear. You might need to repeat the treatment. The main side effects include pain and swelling.
- **Electrocautery**. This procedure uses an electrical current to burn off warts. You might have some pain and swelling after the procedure.
- Surgical excision. Your doctor might use special tools to cut off warts. You'll need local or general **anesthesia** for this treatment, and you might have pain afterward.
- Laser treatments. This approach, which uses an intense beam of light, can be expensive and is usually reserved for extensive and tough-to-treat warts. Side effects can include scarring and pain.

(1010 words)

genital warts 尖锐湿疣

wart [wɔːt] n. [皮肤] 疣(= verruca);[林]
　　树瘤

papilloma [ˌpæpɪˈləumə] n. 乳头状瘤,乳突
　　淋瘤

imiquimod [ɪmɪkwɪˈmɒd] n. 咪喹莫特

podophyllin [ˌpɒdəuˈfɪlɪn] n. 盾叶鬼臼树
　　脂(作泻药用)

podofilox [pəuˈdəfaɪlɒks] n. 普达非洛 (抗

　　有丝分裂药)

trichloroacetic [traɪkləːrəuˈsiːtɪk] n. 三氯
　　乙酰

cryotherapy [ˌkraɪəuˈθerəpi] n. [临床] 冷
　　冻疗法

electrocautery [ɪˌlektrəuˈkɒtəri] n. 电烙
　　器,电烙术

anesthesia [ˌænəsˈθiːziə] n. 麻醉,麻木

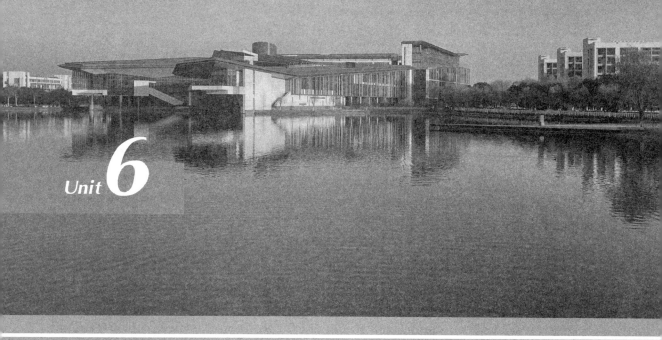

Unit **6**

Some Common Diseases of the Endocrine System

✓参考答案
✓微课等资源

Text A

Diabetes

Diabetes mellitus refers to a group of diseases that affect how your body uses blood sugar (**glucose**). Glucose is vital to your health because it's an important source of energy for the cells that make up your muscles and tissues. It's also your brain's main source of fuel.

The underlying cause of diabetes varies by type. But, no matter what type of diabetes you have, it can lead to excess sugar in your blood. Too much sugar in your blood can lead to serious health problems.

Chronic diabetes conditions include Type 1 diabetes and Type 2 diabetes. Potentially reversible diabetes conditions include **prediabetes** and **gestational** diabetes. Prediabetes occurs when your blood sugar levels are higher than normal, but not high enough to be classified as diabetes. And prediabetes is often the precursor of diabetes unless appropriate measures are taken to prevent progression. Gestational diabetes occurs during pregnancy but may resolve after the baby is delivered.

Symptoms

Diabetes symptoms vary depending on how much your blood sugar is elevated. Some people, especially those with prediabetes or Type 2 diabetes, may sometimes not experience symptoms. In Type 1 diabetes, symptoms tend to come on quickly and be more severe.

Some of the signs and symptoms of Type 1 diabetes and Type 2 diabetes are:

- Increased thirst;
- Frequent urination;
- Extreme hunger;
- Unexplained weight loss;
- Presence of **ketones** in the urine (ketones are a byproduct of the breakdown of muscle and fat that happens when there's not enough available insulin);
- Fatigue;
- Irritability;

- Blurred vision;
- Slow-healing sores;
- Frequent infections, such as gums or skin infections and vaginal infections.

Type 1 diabetes can develop at any age, though it often appears during childhood or adolescence. Type 2 diabetes, the more common type, can develop at any age, though it's more common in people older than 40.

Causes

Causes of Type 1 diabetes

The exact cause of Type 1 diabetes is unknown. What is known is that your immune system—which normally fights harmful bacteria or viruses—attacks and destroys your insulin-producing cells in the pancreas. This leaves you with little or no insulin. Instead of being transported into your cells, sugar builds up in your bloodstream.

Type 1 is thought to be caused by a combination of genetic susceptibility and environmental factors, though exactly what those factors are is still unclear. Weight is not believed to be a factor in Type 1 diabetes.

Causes of prediabetes and Type 2 diabetes

In prediabetes which can lead to Type 2 diabetes and in Type 2 diabetes, your cells become resistant to the action of insulin, and your pancreas is unable to make enough insulin to overcome this resistance. Instead of moving into your cells where it's needed for energy, sugar builds up in your bloodstream.

Exactly why this happens is uncertain, although it's believed that genetic and environmental factors play a role in the development of Type 2 diabetes too. Being overweight is strongly linked to the development of Type 2 diabetes, but not everyone with Type 2 is overweight.

Causes of gestational diabetes

During pregnancy, the **placenta** produces hormones to sustain your pregnancy. These hormones make your cells more resistant to insulin.

Normally, your pancreas responds by producing enough extra insulin to overcome this resistance. But sometimes your pancreas can't keep up. When this happens, too little glucose gets into your cells and too much stays in your blood, resulting in gestational diabetes.

Diagnosis

Symptoms of Type 1 diabetes often appear suddenly and are often the reason for checking blood sugar levels. Symptoms of other types of diabetes and prediabetes come on more gradually or may not be evident.

Tests for Type 1 and Type 2 diabetes and prediabetes

• **Glycated** hemoglobin (A1C) test. This blood test, which doesn't require fasting, indicates your average blood sugar level for the past two to three months.

• Random blood sugar test. A blood sample will be taken at a random time.

• Fasting blood sugar test. A blood sample will be taken after an overnight fast.

• Oral glucose tolerance test. For this test, you fast overnight, and the fasting blood sugar level is measured.

Tests for gestational diabetes

Your doctor may use the following screening tests:

• Initial glucose challenge test. You'll begin the glucose challenge test by drinking a syrupy glucose solution. One hour later, you'll have a blood test to measure your blood sugar level.

• Follow-up glucose tolerance testing. For the follow-up test, you'll be asked to fast overnight and then have your fasting blood sugar level measured. Then you'll drink another sweet solution and your blood sugar level will be checked every hour for a period of three hours.

Treatment

Depending on what type of diabetes you have, blood sugar monitoring, insulin and oral medications may play a role in your treatment. Eating a healthy diet, maintaining a healthy weight and participating in regular activity also are important factors in managing diabetes.

Treatments for Type 1 and Type 2 diabetes

Treatment for Type 1 diabetes involves insulin injections or the use of an insulin pump, frequent blood sugar checks, and carbohydrate counting. Treatment of Type 2 diabetes primarily involves lifestyle changes, monitoring of your blood sugar, along with diabetes medications, insulin or both.

• Monitoring your blood sugar. Depending on your treatment plan, you may check and record your blood sugar as many as four times a day or more often if you're taking insulin.

- Insulin. People with Type 1 diabetes need insulin therapy to survive. Many people with Type 2 diabetes or gestational diabetes also need insulin therapy.

- Oral or other medications. Sometimes other oral or injected medications are prescribed as well.

- Transplantation. In some people who have Type 1 diabetes, a pancreas transplant may be an option.

- **Bariatric** surgery. Although it is not specifically considered a treatment for Type 2 diabetes, people with Type 2 diabetes who are obese and have a body mass index higher than 35 may benefit from this type of surgery.

Treatment for gestational diabetes

Controlling your blood sugar level is essential to keeping your baby healthy and avoiding complications during delivery. In addition to maintaining a healthy diet and exercising, your treatment plan may include monitoring your blood sugar and, in some cases, using insulin or oral medications.

Treatment for prediabetes

If you have prediabetes, healthy lifestyle choices can help you bring your blood sugar level back to normal or at least keep it from rising toward the levels seen in Type 2 diabetes. Maintaining a healthy weight through exercise and healthy eating can help. Exercising at least 150 minutes a week and losing about 7% of your body weight may prevent or delay Type 2 diabetes.

Sometimes medications—such as **metformin** (Glucophage, Glumetza, others)—also are an option if you're at high risk of diabetes, including when your prediabetes is worsening or if you have cardiovascular disease, fatty liver disease or **polycystic ovary syndrome**.

(1166 words)

◇ **Vocabulary**

diabetes mellitus ['melɪtəs] [内科] 糖尿病
glucose ['gluːkəʊs] *n.* 葡萄糖；葡糖
prediabetes ['priːˌdaɪə'biːtiːz] *n.* [内科] 前驱糖尿病

gestational [dʒe'steɪʃənəl] *adj.* 妊娠期的
ketone ['kiːtəʊn] *n.* 酮
placenta [plə'sentə] *n.* [胚] 胎盘；[植] 胎座

glycated ['glaɪkeɪtɪd] *adj.* 糖化的

bariatric [ˌbæɪ'ætrɪks] *adj.* 肥胖症治疗学的

metformin [met'fɔːmɪn] *n.* 二甲双胍（抗糖尿病药、降血糖药）

polycystic ovary syndrome 多囊卵巢综合征

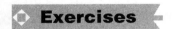 **Exercises**

Ⅰ. **Decide whether the following sentences are *True* or *False* according to the text.**

1. Glucose is an important source of energy for the cells that make up your muscles and tissues.

2. Prediabetes has the same blood sugar levels as Type 1 and 2 diabetes.

3. Gestational diabetes occurs during pregnancy and never resolve even if the baby is delivered.

4. Signs and symptoms of Type 1 and 2 diabetes include increased thirst, frequent urination, extreme hunger, and weight loss, etc.

5. Type 1 diabetes can develop at any age, but Type 2 diabetes only develop among older people.

6. The cause of Type 1 diabetes is known, that is your immune system destroys your insulin-producing cells in the pancreas, resulting in little or no insulin.

7. In prediabetes and Type 2 diabetes, your pancreas is unable to make enough insulin.

8. Tests for Type 1 and Type 2 diabetes include A1C test, fasting blood sugar test, oral glucose tolerance test, etc.

9. Treatment for Type 1 diabetes involves insulin injections, but treatment of Type 2 diabetes primarily involves lifestyle changes.

10. For prediabetes, healthy lifestyle choices can't help you bring your blood sugar level back to normal.

Ⅱ. **Fill in the blanks with the proper form of words in the box.**

gestational	placenta	bariatric	ovary	diabetes
prediabetes	pancreas	hemoglobin	glucose	urinate

1. _____ is a polygenic disease characterized by abnormally high glucose levels in the blood.

2. _____ is a type of sugar that gives you energy.

3. _____ occurs when your blood sugar levels are higher but not high to be classified as diabetes.

4. _____ is the process in which babies grow inside their mother's body before they are born.

5. Your _____ produces insulin and substances that help your body digest food.

6. The _____ is inside the uterus of a pregnant woman, which the unborn baby is attached to.

7. _____ circulates in your blood and they carry oxygen.

8. _____ is of or relating to the treatment of obesity.

9. A woman's _____ are the two organs in her body that produce eggs.

10. Antidiuretic prescriptions can reduce nighttime _____.

Ⅲ. **Translation: translate the passage into Chinese.**

Diabetic retinopathy is the most common form of diabetic eye disease. Diabetic retinopathy usually only affects people who have had diabetes (diagnosed or undiagnosed) for a significant number of years. Retinopathy can affect all diabetics and becomes particularly dangerous, increasing the risk of blindness, if it is left untreated. The risk of developing diabetic retinopathy is known to increase with age as well with less well controlled blood sugar and blood pressure level. According to the NHS, 1,280 new cases of blindness caused by diabetic retinopathy are reported each year in England alone, while a further 4,200 people in the country are thought to be at risk of retinopathy-related vision loss.

All people with diabetes should have a dilated eye examination at least once every year to check for diabetic retinopathy. Diabetic retinopathy includes 3 different types: background retinopathy, diabetic maculopathy, and proliferative retinopathy. The early stages of diabetic retinopathy may occur without symptoms and without pain. An actual influence on the vision will not occur until the disease advances. Symptoms may only become noticeable once the disease advances, but the typical symptoms of retinopathy to look out for include: sudden changes in vision / blurred vision, eye floaters and spots, double vision, eye pain.

Diabetic retinopathy is caused by prolonged high blood glucose levels. Over time, high sugar glucose levels can weaken and damage the small blood vessels within the retina. This may cause haemorrhages, exudates and even swelling of the retina. This then starves the retina of oxygen, and abnormal vessels may grow. Good blood glucose control helps to lower diabetes retinopathy risks.

Laser surgery is often used in the treatment of diabetic eye disease, but each stage of diabetic retinopathy can be treated in a different way. Background retinopathy has no treatment but patients will need regular eye examinations. Maculopathy is usually treated with laser treatment (tiny burns that help to prevent new blood vessel growth and improve the nutrient and oxygen supply to the retina). Proliferative retinopathy is also treated with lasers, with a scattering over the whole retina. This destroys the starved area of the retina. Serious diabetes retinopathy cases may require eye surgery.

(359 words)

Ⅳ. Give a presentation.

Dictate the causes, symptoms, treatments, etc. of Diabetes in English with 3—4 students. Try to use the formal expression, especially related medical terminology when you make your presentation.

Ⅴ. Write a certificate of sick leave.

根据下列内容,写一份病假证明。

张虹,35 岁,高烧 39℃,连续咳嗽一周,乏力,头痛,四肢疼痛。建议在家休息一周,用药三天后来院复查。上海人民医院医生王英亮,2019 年 5 月 9 日。

Text B

Hyperthyroidism

Hyperthyroidism (overactive thyroid) occurs when your thyroid gland produces too much of the hormone **thyroxine**. Hyperthyroidism can accelerate your body's metabolism, causing unintentional weight loss and a rapid or irregular heartbeat.

Several treatments are available for hyperthyroidism. Doctors use anti-thyroid medications and radioactive **iodine** to slow the production of thyroid hormones. Sometimes, hyperthyroidism treatment involves surgery to remove all or part of your thyroid gland.

Although hyperthyroidism can be serious if you ignore it, most people respond well once hyperthyroidism is diagnosed and treated.

Symptoms

Hyperthyroidism can **mimic** other health problems, which can make it difficult for your doctor to diagnose. It can also cause a wide variety of signs and symptoms, including:

- Unintentional weight loss, even when your appetite and food intake stay the same or increase;
- Rapid heartbeat (**tachycardia**)—commonly more than 100 beats a minute;
- Irregular heartbeat (arrhythmia);
- Pounding of your heart (palpitations);
- Increased appetite;
- Nervousness, anxiety and irritability;
- **Tremor**—usually a fine trembling in your hands and fingers;
- Sweating;
- Changes in menstrual patterns;
- Increased sensitivity to heat;
- Changes in bowel patterns, especially more frequent bowel movements;
- An enlarged thyroid gland (**goiter**), which may appear as a swelling at the base of your neck;
- Fatigue, muscle weakness;
- Difficulty sleeping;

- Skin thinning;
- Fine, brittle hair.

Older adults are more likely to have either no signs or symptoms or subtle ones, such as an increased heart rate, heat intolerance and a tendency to become tired during ordinary activities.

Causes

Hyperthyroidism can be caused by a number of conditions, including Graves' disease, Plummer's disease and **thyroiditis**.

Your thyroid is a small, butterfly-shaped gland at the base of your neck, just below your **Adam's apple**. The thyroid gland has an enormous impact on your health. Every aspect of your metabolism is regulated by thyroid hormones.

Your thyroid gland produces two main hormones, thyroxine (T4) and **triiodothyronine** (T3), that influence every cell in your body. They maintain the rate at which your body uses fats and carbohydrates, help control your body temperature, influence your heart rate, and help regulate the production of protein. Your thyroid also produces a hormone that helps regulate the amount of calcium in your blood (**calcitonin**).

Reasons for too much thyroxine (T4)

Normally, your thyroid releases the right amount of hormones, but sometimes it produces too much T4. This may occur for a number of reasons, including:

- Graves' disease. Graves' disease is an autoimmune disorder in which antibodies produced by your immune system stimulate your thyroid to produce too much T4. It's the most common cause of hyperthyroidism.
- Hyperfunctioning thyroid **nodules**. This form of hyperthyroidism occurs when one or more **adenomas** of your thyroid produce too much T4. An adenoma is a part of the gland that has walled itself off from the rest of the gland, forming noncancerous (benign) lumps that may cause an enlargement of the thyroid.
- Thyroiditis. Sometimes your thyroid gland can become inflamed after pregnancy, due to an autoimmune condition or for unknown reasons. The inflammation can cause excess thyroid hormone stored in the gland to leak into your bloodstream. Some types of thyroiditis may cause pain, while others are painless.

Diagnosis

Hyperthyroidism is diagnosed using:

• Medical history and physical exam. During the exam your doctor may try to detect a slight tremor in your fingers when they're extended, overactive reflexes, eye changes and warm, moist skin. Your doctor will also examine your thyroid gland as you swallow to see if it's enlarged, bumpy or tender and check your pulse to see if it's rapid or irregular.

• Blood tests. Blood tests that measure thyroxine and thyroid-stimulating hormone (TSH) can confirm the diagnosis. High levels of thyroxine and low or nonexistent amounts of TSH indicate an overactive thyroid. The amount of TSH is important because it's the hormone that signals your thyroid gland to produce more thyroxine.

If blood tests indicate hyperthyroidism, your doctor may recommend one of the following tests to help determine why your thyroid is overactive:

• **Radioiodine** uptake test. For this test, you take a small, oral dose of radioactive iodine (radioiodine) to see how much will collect in your thyroid gland. You'll be checked after 4, 6 or 24 hours—and sometimes after all three time periods—to see how much iodine your thyroid has absorbed.

• Thyroid scan. During this test, you'll have a radioactive **isotope** injected into the vein on the inside of your elbow or sometimes into a vein in your hand. You then lie on a table with your head stretched backward while a special camera produces an image of your thyroid gland on a computer screen. This test shows how iodine collects in your thyroid.

• Thyroid ultrasound. This test uses high-frequency sound waves to produce images of the thyroid. Ultrasound may be better at detecting thyroid nodules than other tests, and there's no exposure to any radiation.

Treatment

Several treatments for hyperthyroidism exist. The best approach for you depends on your age, physical condition, the underlying cause of the hyperthyroidism, personal preference and the severity of your disorder. Possible treatments include:

• Radioactive iodine. Taken by mouth, radioactive iodine is absorbed by your thyroid gland, where it causes the gland to shrink. Symptoms usually subside within several months. Excess radioactive iodine disappears from the body in weeks to months.

• Anti-thyroid medications. These medications gradually reduce symptoms of hyperthyroidism by preventing your thyroid gland from producing excess amounts of hormones. They include **methimazole** (Tapazole) and propylithiouracil. Symptoms usually begin to improve within several weeks to months, but treatment with anti-thyroid medications typically continues at least a year and often longer.

• Beta blockers. Although these drugs are usually used to treat high blood pressure and don't affect thyroid levels, they can ease symptoms of hyperthyroidism, such as a tremor, rapid heart rate and palpitations. For that reason, your doctor may prescribe them to help you feel better until your thyroid levels are closer to normal. These medications generally aren't recommended for people who have asthma, and side effects may include fatigue and sexual dysfunction.

• Surgery (**thyroidectomy**). If you're pregnant or you otherwise can't tolerate anti-thyroid drugs and don't want to or can't have radioactive iodine therapy, you may be a candidate for thyroid surgery, although this is an option in only a few cases.

In a thyroidectomy, your doctor removes most of your thyroid gland. Risks of this surgery include damage to your vocal cords and **parathyroid** glands—four tiny glands situated on the back of your thyroid gland that help control the level of calcium in your blood.

(1112 words)

◆ **Vocabulary**

hyperthyroidism [ˌhaɪpə'θaɪrɔɪdɪzəm] n. 甲状腺功能亢进

thyroxine [θaɪ'rɒksiːn] n. [生化] 甲状腺素

iodine ['aɪədiːn] n. 碘, 碘酒

mimic ['mɪmɪk] v. 模仿, 模拟; (疾病) 表现出 (另一种疾病) 的症状

tachycardia [ˌtækɪ'kɑːdɪə] n. [内科] 心动过速, 心跳过速

tremor ['tremə(r)] n. 震动, 颤动

goiter ['gɔɪtər] n. 甲状腺肿

thyroiditis [ˌθaɪrɔɪ'daɪtɪs] n. [内科] 甲状腺炎

Adam's apple 喉结

triiodothyronine [traɪaɪədəʊ'θaɪrənin] n. [药] 碘塞罗宁

calcitonin [ˌkælsɪ'təʊnɪn] n. [生化] 降血钙素 (等于 thyrocalcitonin)

nodule ['nɒdjuːl] n. [医] 小瘤, 小结节

adenoma [ˌædə'nəʊmə] n. 腺瘤

radioiodine [ˌreɪdɪəʊ'aɪəʊdiːn] n. [特医] [核] 放射碘

isotope ['aɪsətəʊp] n. 同位素

methimazole [me'θaɪməzəʊl] n. 甲巯咪唑, [药] 甲巯基咪唑 (抗甲状腺药)

thyroidectomy [ˌθaɪrɔɪˈdektəmi] n. [外科]
甲状腺切除术

parathyroid [ˌpærəˈθaɪrɔɪd] adj. 副甲状腺
的 n. 甲状旁腺

◇ **Exercises**

Ⅰ. **Decide whether the following sentences are *True* or *False* according to the text.**

1. Hyperthyroidism can accelerate body's metabolism, resulting in weight loss and rapid heartbeat.

2. Hyperthyroidism treatment involves using anti-thyroid medications, radioactive iodine, etc.

3. Hyperthyroidism occurs when your thyroid gland produces less hormone thyroxine.

4. Tachycardia, palpitations, and sweating are the signs and symptoms of hyperthyroidism.

5. Older people with hyperthyroidism are more likely to have signs and symptoms.

6. Hyperthyroidism can be caused by Graves' disease, Plummer's disease and thyroiditis.

7. If blood tests indicate hyperthyroidism, your doctor may recommend thyroid scan to find the causes.

8. The thyroid is a butterfly-shaped gland, just above your Adam's apple.

9. Hyperthyroidism can mimic other health problems, but it's easier for doctors to diagnose.

10. The thyroid gland can produces T4, T3 and a hormone which regulates the calcium in the blood.

Ⅱ. **Fill in the blanks with the proper form of words in the box.**

tremor	thyroidectomy	nodule	isotope	arrhythmia
thyroxine	tachycardia	hyperthyroidism	adenoma	goiter

1. _____ is a hormone produced by the thyroid glands to regulate metabolism by controlling the rate of oxidation in cells.

2. _____ is an overactive thyroid gland, causing nervousness, insomnia, sweating, and palpitation.

3. _____ refers to the abnormally rapid heartbeat (over 100 beats per minute).

4. An abnormal rate of muscle contractions in the heart is called _____.

5. A _____ is a shaking of your body or voice that you cannot control.

6. _____ is a disease of the thyroid gland that makes a person's neck very swollen.

7. A _____ is a small round lump that can appear on your body and is a sign of an illness.

8. _____ is a tumour, usually benign, occurring in glandular tissue.

9. Surgical removal of all or part of the thyroid gland is called _____.

10. _____ are atoms that have the same number of protons and electrons but different numbers of neutrons and therefore have different physical properties.

Ⅲ. **Translation: translate the passage into Chinese.**

Hypothyroidism, or underactive thyroid, happens when your thyroid gland doesn't make enough thyroid hormones to meet your body's needs. Your thyroid is a small, butterfly-shaped gland in the front of your neck. It makes hormones that control the way the body uses energy. These hormones affect nearly every organ in your body and control many of your body's most important functions. For example, they affect your breathing, heart rate, weight, digestion, and moods. Without enough thyroid hormones, many of your body's functions slow down. But there are treatments that can help.

Hypothyroidism has several causes. They include Hashimoto's disease (an autoimmune disorder where your immune system attacks your thyroid. This is the most common cause), thyroiditis (inflammation of the thyroid), congenital hypothyroidism (hypothyroidism that is present at birth), surgical removal of part or all of the thyroid, radiation treatment of the thyroid, certain medicines.

The symptoms of hypothyroidism can vary from person to person and may include fatigue, weight gain, a puffy face, trouble tolerating cold, joint and muscle pain, constipation, dry skin, thinning hair, decreased sweating, heavy or irregular menstrual periods, fertility problems in women, depression, slowed heart rate. Because hypothyroidism develops slowly, many people don't notice symptoms of the disease for months or even years.

The treatment for hypothyroidism is medicine to replace the hormone that your own thyroid can no longer make. About 6 to 8 weeks after you start taking the medicine, you will get a blood test to check your thyroid hormone level. Your health care provider will adjust your dose if needed. Each time your dose is adjusted, you'll have another blood test. Once you find the right dose, you will probably get a blood test in 6 months. After that, you will need the test once a year. If you take your medicine according to the instructions, you usually should be able to control the hypothyroidism. You should never stop taking your medicine without talking with your health care provider first. If you have Hashimoto's disease or other types of autoimmune thyroid disorders, you may be sensitive to harmful side effects from iodine. Talk to your health care provider about which foods, supplements, and medicines you need to avoid. Women need more iodine when they are pregnant because the baby gets iodine from the mother's diet. If you are pregnant, talk with your health care provider about how much iodine you need.

(399 words)

IV. Give a presentation.

Dictate the causes, symptoms, treatments, etc. of Hyperthyroidism in English with 3—4 students. Try to use the formal expression, especially related medical terminology when you make your presentation.

V. Write a vaccination certificate.

根据下列内容，写一份接种证明。

张一鸣，女，20 岁，今年已接种乙肝疫苗。广州市红十字会医院医疗保健中心主治医生张雪莲，2021 年 6 月 7 日。

Text C

Thyroiditis

Thyroiditis is a swelling of your thyroid gland. It mostly affects women from early adulthood to middle age, but anyone can get it. The thyroid is the butterfly-shaped gland in the front of your throat, just below your Adam's apple. It controls your metabolism by making hormones that influence how fast or slow your heart, brain, and other parts of your body work.

There are different types of thyroiditis, but they all cause inflammation and swelling of your thyroid. They can make it produce too many or not enough hormones. Too many can make you feel **jittery** and possibly make your heart race. Too few and you may feel tired and depressed.

About 20 million Americans have a form of thyroid disease. Like the others, thyroiditis can be a serious illness. Treatment will depend on the type you have and the symptoms it causes.

Thyroiditis has three phases:

• **Thyrotoxic** phase. The thyroid is swollen and releases too many hormones.

• **Hypothyroid** phase. After a few weeks or months, too much of the thyroid hormone is released and leads to hypothyroidism, when you don't have enough left.

• **Euthyroid** phase. In this phase, thyroid levels are normal. It can happen between the first two phases or at the end, after the swelling has gone down.

Symptoms

Common symptoms include fatigue, swelling at the base of your neck, and sometimes some pain in the front of your throat. However, other symptoms will vary, depending on whether your thyroid is underactive (hypothyroidism) or overactive (hyperthyroidism).

Symptoms of hypothyroidism may include:

• Fatigue;
• Depression;
• Weight gain;

- Dry skin;
- Constipation;
- Muscle aches;
- Intolerance to cold.

Symptoms of hyperthyroidism may include:

- Anxiety and irritability;
- Weight loss;
- Insomnia;
- Heart palpitations;
- Muscle weakness;
- Intolerance to heat.

Causes and types

Many things can make your thyroid swell. You may have gotten an infection from a virus or bacteria. You may be taking a drug like **lithium** or interferon. Or you may have problems with your immune system. One form of thyroiditis shows up after childbirth. Pregnancy has a major impact on the thyroid in general.

These are the most common causes:

• **Hashimoto's disease**. This is the most common type of thyroiditis. Your immune system attacks your thyroid and slowly weakens the gland until it can't make enough thyroid hormones.

• Subacute thyroiditis. This type is often triggered by an infection. There's usually a pattern of how the thyroid functions. First, the thyroid and neck area are painful. Then, the thyroid makes too much hormone, called hyperthyroidism. Then, your thyroid works normally, followed by a time where the thyroid produces too little thyroid hormone. This is called hypothyroidism. After about 12 to 18 months, thyroid function returns to normal.

• **Postpartum** thyroiditis. This type begins within a year after childbirth, particularly in women with a history of thyroid issues. With treatment, the thyroid usually recovers within 18 months.

• Silent thyroiditis. As the name suggests, there are no symptoms with this type. It's similar to postpartum thyroiditis, and recovery usually takes up to 18 months. It starts with a phase of too much hormone production, followed by a longer period of the thyroid making too little.

Diagnosis

Your doctor may give you one or more of these tests.

• Blood test. Thyroid hormones circulate in your blood, and their levels can help your doctor figure out the specific kind of thyroiditis you have.

• Radioactive iodine uptake test (RAIU). Because iodine collects in your thyroid gland, a doctor or nurse gives you radioactive iodine as a pill or liquid. Over the next 24 hours, your doctor will check at several points to see how much iodine your thyroid has absorbed.

• Thyroid scan. You get a shot of radioactive iodine. You lie face up on a table with your head bent back, exposing your neck. Your doctor uses a device to take images of your thyroid.

• **Erythrocyte sedimentation** rate (ESR or sed rate). This test measures swelling by how fast your red blood cells fall. High ESR may mean you have subacute thyroiditis.

• Ultrasound. A **sonogram** of your thyroid can show a nodule or growth, a change in blood flow, and the texture or density of the gland.

Treatment

Treatment depends on the type of thyroiditis you have.

Doctors usually treat hypothyroidism with synthetic versions of thyroid hormone. They come in pills that you swallow. As your metabolism returns to normal, your doctor may adjust the dosage.

The treatment of hyperthyroidism depends on the type of inflammation and on any symptoms you have.

Beta-blockers often treat symptoms like a fast heart rate and palpitations. Antithyroid medicines can lower the amount of hormones that your thyroid is making. Sometimes, your doctor may prescribe a form of radioactive iodine to shrink the thyroid and reduce any symptoms.

If you have thyroid pain, your doctor may recommend nothing more than aspirin or ibuprofen. Severe pain may be treated in other ways.

It's rare, but you may need surgery if other treatments don't work.

(861 words)

◈ Vocabulary

thyroiditis [θaɪrɔɪˈdaɪtɪs] *n.* 甲状腺炎

jittery [ˈdʒɪtəri] *adj.* 神经过敏的，紧张不安的

thyrotoxic [θaɪrəʊˈtɒksɪk] *adj.* 甲状腺毒性的

hypothyroid [ˌhaɪpəʊˈθaɪrɔɪd] *adj.* 甲状腺机能减退的

euthyroid [juːˈθaɪərɔɪd] *adj.* 甲状腺机能正常的

lithium [ˈlɪθɪəm] *n.* 锂

Hashimoto's disease 桥本氏病，慢性甲状腺炎（= Hashimoto's thyroiditis）

postpartum [pəʊstˈpɑːtəm] *adj.* 产后的，产后用的

erythrocyte [ɪˈrɪθrəsaɪt] *n.* [细胞] 红细胞

sedimentation [ˌsedimenˈteɪʃn] *n.* 沉积（作用）

sonogram [ˈsəʊnəɡræm] *n.* 声波图，声谱记录，语图

Text D

Primary Aldosteronism

Primary **aldosteronism** is a hormonal disorder that leads to high blood pressure. It occurs when your adrenal glands produce too much of a hormone called aldosterone. Your adrenal glands produce a number of essential hormones, including aldosterone. Usually, aldosterone balances sodium and potassium in your blood. But too much of this hormone can cause you to lose potassium and retain sodium. That imbalance can cause your body to hold too much water, increasing your blood volume and blood pressure. Treatment options include medications, surgery and lifestyle changes.

Symptoms

Primary aldosteronism often doesn't cause clear symptoms. The first clue that you may have primary aldosteronism is usually high blood pressure, especially hard to control blood pressure. Sometimes, primary aldosteronism causes low potassium levels. If this happens, you may have:

- Muscle cramps;
- Fatigue;
- Excessive thirst;
- Weakness;
- Headache;
- A frequent need to urinate.

Causes

Common conditions that can cause too much aldosterone include:

- A benign growth in an adrenal gland;
- Overactivity of both adrenal glands.

There are other, much rarer causes of primary aldosteronism, including:

- A cancerous growth on the outer layer of the adrenal gland;
- An inherited condition that causes high blood pressure in children and young adults.

Complications

Primary aldosteronism can lead to high blood pressure and low potassium levels. These complications in turn can lead to other problems.

Problems related to high blood pressure

Persistently elevated blood pressure can lead to problems with your heart and kidneys, including:

- Heart attack, heart failure and other heart problems;
- Stroke;
- Kidney disease or kidney failure.

People with primary aldosteronism have a higher than expected risk of cardiovascular problems compared with people who only have high blood pressure.

*Problems related to low potassium levels (**hypokalemia**)*

Primary aldosteronism may cause low potassium levels. If your potassium levels are just slightly low, you may not have any symptoms. Very low levels of potassium can lead to:

- Weakness;
- Muscle cramps;
- Irregular heart rhythm;
- Excess thirst or urination.

Diagnosis

If your doctor suspects primary aldosteronism, you'll likely have a test to measure levels of aldosterone and renin in your blood. Renin is an enzyme released by your kidneys that helps control blood pressure. If your renin level is very low and your aldosterone level is high, you may have primary aldosteronism.

Additional tests

If the aldosterone-renin test suggests primary aldosteronism, you'll need other tests to confirm the diagnosis and look for potential causes. Possible tests include:

- Salt-loading test. There are a few ways to do this blood or urine test. You may eat a high-sodium diet for a few days or you could have a saline infusion for several hours before your doctor measures your aldosterone levels. You may also be given fludrocortisone—a drug that mimics the action of aldosterone—in addition to the high-sodium diet before the test.
- Abdominal CT scan. A CT scan may find a tumor on your adrenal gland or show an enlarged adrenal gland that suggests the gland is overactive.
- Adrenal vein blood test. A radiologist draws blood from both your right and left adrenal veins and compares the two samples. If only one side has elevated aldosterone, your doctor may suspect a growth on that adrenal

gland.

This test involves placing a tube in a vein in your **groin** and threading it up to the adrenal veins. Though essential for determining the appropriate treatment, this test carries the risk of bleeding or a blood clot in the vein.

Treatment

Treatment for primary aldosteronism depends on the underlying cause. The basic goal is to get your aldosterone levels back to normal or to block the effect of high aldosterone to prevent complications.

Treatment for an adrenal gland tumor

An adrenal gland tumor may be treated with surgery or medications and lifestyle changes.

• Surgical removal of the gland. Surgical removal of the adrenal gland with the tumor (**adrenalectomy**) is usually recommended. Surgical removal may bring blood pressure, potassium and aldosterone levels back to normal. Your doctor will follow you closely after surgery and progressively adjust or eliminate your high blood pressure medications. Risks of surgery include bleeding and infection. Adrenal hormone replacement isn't necessary because the other adrenal gland can make enough of all the hormones your body needs.

• Aldosterone-blocking drugs. If your primary aldosteronism is caused by a benign tumor and you can't have surgery or prefer not to, you can be treated with aldosterone-blocking drugs called **mineralocorticoid** receptor antagonists (**spironolactone** and **eplerenone**) and lifestyle changes. High blood pressure and low potassium will return if you stop taking your medications.

Treatment for overactivity of both adrenal glands

A combination of medications and lifestyle modifications can effectively treat primary aldosteronism caused by overactivity of both adrenal glands.

• Medications. Mineralocorticoid receptor antagonists block the action of aldosterone in your body. Your doctor may first prescribe spironolactone (Aldactone). This medication helps correct high blood pressure and low potassium, but may cause other problems.

In addition to blocking aldosterone receptors, spironolactone may inhibit the action of other hormones. Side effects can include male breast enlargement (**gynecomastia**) and menstrual irregularities in women.

A newer, more-expensive mineralocorticoid receptor antagonist called eplerenone (Inspra) eliminates the sex hormone side effects associated with spironolactone. Your doctor may recommend eplerenone if you have serious side effects with spironolactone. You may also need other medications for high blood pressure.

• Lifestyle changes. High blood pressure medications are more effective when combined with a healthy diet and lifestyle. Work with your doctor to create a plan to lower the sodium in your diet and keep a healthy body weight. Getting regular exercise, limiting the amount of alcohol you drink and stopping smoking also may improve your response to medications.

Lifestyle and home remedies

A healthy lifestyle is essential for keeping blood pressure low and keeping long-term heart health. Here are some healthy lifestyle suggestions:

• Eat a healthy diet. Diets that highlight a healthy variety of foods—including grains, fruits, vegetables and low-fat dairy products—can help with weight loss and help lower blood pressure.

• Achieve a healthy weight. If your body mass index (BMI) is 25 or more, losing as little as 3% to 5% of your body weight may lower your blood pressure.

• Exercise. Regular aerobic exercise can help lower blood pressure. Taking a moderately paced walk for 30 minutes most days of the week can improve your health.

• Don't smoke. Quitting smoking improves your overall heart and blood vessel health.

(1088 words)

◈ **Vocabulary**

aldosteronism [ˌældəʊˈsterənɪzəm] *n.* [内科] 醛甾酮增多症

primary aldosteronism 原发性醛固酮增多症

hypokalemia [ˌhaɪpəʊkeɪˈliːmjə] *n.* 低钾血，血钾过少

groin [ɡrɔɪn] *n.* [解剖] 腹股沟

adrenalectomy [əˌdrɪnəˈlektəmi] *n.* [泌尿] 肾上腺切除术

mineralocorticoid [mɪnərələˈkɔːrtɪkɔɪd] *n.* 盐皮质激素

spironolactone [ˌspaɪrənəʊˈlæktəʊn] *n.* [药] 螺内酯

eplerenone [ˈɪplərɪnən] *n.* [药] 依普利酮

gynecomastia [dʒɪnɪkəʊˈmæstɪə] *adj.* [内科] 男子女性型乳房

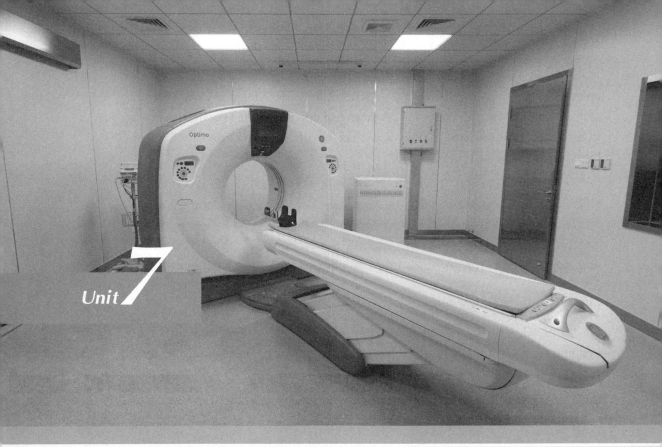

Unit 7

Some Common Diseases of the Nervous System

✓参考答案
✓微课等资源

Text A

Subarachnoid Hemorrhage

A **subarachnoid hemorrhage** is a type of bleeding stroke that happens between your brain and the **membrane** that surrounds it. (This area is called the "subarachnoid" space; "hemorrhage" means bleeding.) It can happen when an artery is damaged and starts to bleed.

Symptoms

Like any other stroke, a subarachnoid hemorrhage is an emergency. Call the emergency number 911 (in the west) or 120 (in China) right away if you suspect you or anyone close to you has had one. It may feel like the worst headache you've ever had. Symptoms may also include:

- Nausea, vomiting, or both;
- Stiff neck or neck pain;
- Back pain;
- Double vision;
- Problems talking;
- Drooping eyelid;
- Confusion;
- Dizziness;
- Light sensitivity;
- Seizures;
- Passing out;
- Weakness on one side of the body or other stroke-like symptoms;
- Loss of alertness.

Don't delay—call the emergency number right away.

Causes

A subarachnoid hemorrhage happens most often when there's a bulge in an artery wall near the surface of the brain. Other causes include:

- Bleeding from an **arteriovenous** malformation (AVM), an abnormal tangle of blood vessels in the brain;
- Other blood vessel issues;

- A head injury, such as from a car accident or fall.

Risk factors

It's not possible to prevent all subarachnoid hemorrhages. But if aneurysms run in your family, tell your doctor. You may need to get tested to find out if you have a brain aneurysm that hasn't ruptured. These things also raise your risk for a subarachnoid hemorrhage:

- High blood pressure;
- Cigarette smoking;
- **Methamphetamine** or cocaine use;
- Heavy drinking of alcohol.

They're also slightly more common in women.

Diagnosis

You may get one or more of these imaging tests to see if there's bleeding in your brain:

CT scan. Computed tomography uses a series of X-rays combined by a computer to form an image that's more detailed than a single X-ray. You may get a contrast dye by IV to provide better images. A CT scan doesn't always show a small subarachnoid hemorrhage or one that happened a week or more ago.

MRI. Magnetic resonance imaging uses a large magnet and radio waves to create images of your brain. You might get a contrast dye by IV to enhance the images. It can reveal bleeding that's happened in the recent past.

Other tests that can help with diagnosis include:

- Cerebral **angiogram**. You'll have a catheter (a thin, flexible tube) placed into an artery in your leg and threaded up to your brain. Then you'll get a contrast dye by IV to highlight the blood vessels in your brain on X-rays.
- Spinal tap. Also called a lumbar puncture, a health care worker will put a needle into your back to collect spinal fluid to check for blood.
- **Transcranial** ultrasound. This type of ultrasound measures blood flow in your brain.

You may need to repeat imaging tests, such as the CT scan, because bleeding doesn't always show up right away.

Treatment

If you have a subarachnoid hemorrhage, you'll be hospitalized right away, preferably at a center that treats strokes. At the hospital, you may get medications to ease your headache and to help prevent seizures and clot-related ("**ischemic**") strokes that can happen when an artery is blocked. Doctors will try to keep your blood pressure high enough to keep blood flowing in your brain but low enough to stop excessive bleeding. If you have too much fluid in the brain, doctors may need to put in a **shunt**. This thin, flexible tube drains the extra fluid and prevents pressure on the brain.

If you have an aneurysm that has burst, you may get one of the following procedures to stop or prevent further bleeding:

• **Endovascular** coiling. Using the catheter in a cerebral angiogram, your doctor will put a tiny coiled wire into the aneurysm, where it forms a clot that stops the bleeding.

• Endovascular stent. Instead of a coil, you'll get a tiny tube called a stent placed across the aneurysm. The stent channels the blood away from the aneurysm to prevent it from leaking or bursting.

• Clip. Your doctor will make a surgical cut (incision) in your **scalp** and remove a piece of your skull to reach the aneurysm. A special microscope will help your doctor find the aneurysm and fasten a tiny clip across it, replace the piece of skull, and sew up the surgical cut.

• Vessel bypass. A surgeon will attach a blood vessel to the artery past the aneurysm to ensure good blood flow in the brain, once the aneurysm has been repaired. The bypass artery may come from inside of your brain or scalp, or from your arm or leg.

• Endovascular embolization. A surgeon threads a catheter to your brain through an artery in your groin. Coils placed in the aneurysm through the catheter form a clot that stops bleeding.

Complications

A subarachnoid hemorrhage can have serious short-and long-term effects. One potentially fatal problem is that a brain aneurysm will bleed again. This can happen shortly after the first episode of bleeding. Other early problems include **vasospasm** and **hydrocephalus**. Vasospasm happens when a blood vessel narrows and cuts off oxygen to your brain. Hydrocephalus is a buildup of fluid on the brain.

Long-term complications can include seizures and problems with memory and thinking, as well as depression, anxiety, and **posttraumatic** stress disorder (PTSD).

(938 words)

◆ Vocabulary

subarachnoid [ˌsʌbəˈræknɔɪd] *adj.* 蛛网膜下的

hemorrhage [ˈhemərɪdʒ] *n.* 出血（= haemorrhage）

membrane [ˈmembreɪn] *n.* 膜，薄膜；羊皮纸

arteriovenous [ɑːtɪəriːəuviːˈnaʊs] *adj.* 动静脉的

methamphetamine [ˌmeθæmˈfetəmiːn] *n.* 甲基苯丙胺,脱氧麻黄碱（中枢兴奋药）

angiogram [ˈændʒɪəˌɡræm] *n.* 血管造影片

transcranial [trænskˈræniəl] *adj.* 经颅的

ischemic [ɪsˈkiːmɪk] *adj.* 缺血性的,局部缺血的

shunt [ʃʌnt] *n.* 分流管；吻合分流术 *v.* 使……分流

endovascular [ˌendəuˈvæskjʊlə] *adj.* ［医］血管内的

scalp [skælp] *n.* 头皮；战利品

vasospasm [ˈveɪzəuˌspæzəm] *n.* 血管痉挛

hydrocephalus [ˌhaɪdrəuˈsefələs] *n.* ［内科］脑积水

posttraumatic [ˌpəustˌtrɔːˈmætɪk] *adj.* 外伤后的

◆ Exercises

Ⅰ. **Decide whether the following sentences are *True* or *False* according to the text.**

1. A subarachnoid hemorrhage can happen when an artery in "subarachnoid" space is damaged and starts to bleed.

2. A subarachnoid hemorrhage is an emergent stroke and the patient should be sent to hospital at once.

3. Symptoms of a subarachnoid hemorrhage may include double vision and nausea, but headache is excluded.

4. AVM or a head injury can cause subarachnoid hemorrhage.

5. Hypertension and heavy drinking of alcohol are the risk factors for a subarachnoid hemorrhage.

6. CT scan, MRI and cerebral angiogram can help to diagnose a subarachnoid hemorrhage.

7. If someone has a subarachnoid hemorrhage suddenly, he can save himself at home.

8. Endovascular coiling and clip can stop or prevent further bleeding caused by an aneurysm.

9. A subarachnoid hemorrhage can only have serious short-term effects.

10. A CT scan can always show a small subarachnoid hemorrhage or one that happened in the past.

Ⅱ. **Fill in the blanks with the proper form of words in the box.**

endovascular	spasm	arteriovenous	subarachnoid	cerebral
aneurysm	hemorrhage	membrane	malformation	angiogram

1. _____ is an affliction in which some part of the body is misshapen or malformed.

2. Shortly after his admission into the hospital, he had a massive brain _____ and died.

3. A brain _____ is a weak or thin area along an artery wall in the brain.

4. _____ is an X-ray representation of blood vessels made after the injection of a radiopaque substance.

5. A vibrating _____ in the ear helps to convey sounds to the brain.

6. The patient has suffered a type of stroke called _____ hemorrhage (SAH).

7. Cerebral aneurysm and _____ malformation are frequent diseases of cerebral vessels.

8. The _____ convulses her facial muscles.

9. The patient underwent _____ repair under general anesthesia.

10. _____ is of or relating to the cerebrum or brain.

Ⅲ. **Translation: translate the passage into Chinese.**

A migraine is a headache that can cause severe throbbing pain or a pulsing sensation, usually on one side of the head. It's often accompanied by nausea, vomiting, and extreme sensitivity to light and sound. Migraine attacks can last for hours to days, and the pain can be so severe that it interferes with your daily activities. Medications can help prevent some migraines and make them less painful. Migraines, which affect children and teenagers as well as adults, can progress through four stages: prodrome, aura, attack and post-drome. Not everyone who has migraines goes through all stages.

Though migraine causes aren't fully understood, genetics and environmental factors appear to play a role. There are a number of migraine triggers, including:

• Hormonal changes in women. Fluctuations in estrogen, such as before or during menstrual periods, pregnancy and menopause, seem to trigger headaches in many women.

- Hormonal medications, such as oral contraceptives, also can worsen migraines. Some women, however, find that their migraines occur less often when taking these medications.

- Drinks. These include alcohol, especially wine, and too much caffeine, such as coffee.

- Stress. Stress at work or home can cause migraines.

- Sensory stimuli. Bright or flashing lights can induce migraines, as can loud sounds. Strong smells—such as perfume, paint thinner, second-hand smoke and others—trigger migraines in some people.

- Sleep changes. Missing sleep or getting too much sleep can trigger migraines in some people.

- Physical factors. Intense physical exertion, including sexual activity, might provoke migraines.

- Weather changes. A change of weather or barometric pressure can prompt a migraine.

- Medications. Oral contraceptives and vasodilators, such as nitroglycerin, can aggravate migraines.

- Foods. Aged cheeses and salty and processed foods might trigger migraines. So might skipping meals.

- Food additives. These include the sweetener aspartame and the preservative monosodium glutamate (MSG), found in many foods.

(314 words)

IV. Give a presentation.

Dictate the causes, symptoms, treatments, etc. of Subarachnoid Hemorrhage in English with 3—4 students. Try to use the formal expression, especially related medical terminology when you make your presentation.

V. Describe the present illness in English.

根据下列内容,用英语描述疾病症状。

病人神志清醒但语速慢,颅骨和面部正常,瞳孔正常,对光反射敏感,甲状腺未见增大。脉搏 110 次/分,心律不齐,心脏有杂音。

Text B

Parkinson's Disease

Parkinson's disease mostly affects older people but can also occur in younger adults. The symptoms are the result of the gradual degeneration of nerve cells in the portion of the midbrain that controls body movements. The first signs are likely to be barely noticeable—a feeling of weakness or stiffness in one limb, or a fine trembling of one hand when it is at rest. Eventually, the shaking (tremor) worsens and spreads, muscles become stiffer, movements slow down, and balance and coordination deteriorate. As the disease progresses, depression, cognitive issues, and other mental or emotional problems are common.

Parkinson's disease usually begins between the ages of 50 and 65, striking about 1% of the population in that age group; it is slightly more common in men than in women. Medication can treat its symptoms and decrease the disability.

Causes

Body movements are regulated by a portion of the brain called the **basal ganglia**, whose cells require a proper balance of two substances called **dopamine** and **acetylcholine**, both involved in the transmission of nerve impulses. In Parkinson's, cells that produce dopamine begin to degenerate, throwing off the balance of these two **neurotransmitters**. Researchers believe that genetics sometimes plays a role in this cellular breakdown. In rare instances, Parkinson's disease may be caused by a viral infection or by exposure to environmental toxins such as **pesticides**, **carbon monoxide**, or the metal **manganese**. But in the great majority of Parkinson's cases, the cause is unknown. Other causes of **parkinsonism** include:

- An adverse reaction to prescription drugs;
- Use of illegal drugs;
- Exposure to environmental toxins;
- Stroke;
- Thyroid and parathyroid disorders;
- Repeated head trauma (for example, the trauma associated with boxing and multiple **concussions**);

- Brain tumor;
- An excess of fluid around the brain (called hydrocephalus);
- Brain inflammation (**encephalitis**) resulting from infection.

Parkinsonism may also be present in persons with other **neurological** conditions, including Alzheimer's disease, Wilson's disease, and Huntington's disease.

Symptoms

Parkinson's disease is a movement disorder that progresses slowly. Some people will first notice a sense of weakness, difficulty walking, and stiff muscles. Others may notice a tremor of the head or hands. Parkinson's is a progressive disorder and the symptoms gradually worsen. The general symptoms of Parkinson's disease include:

- Slowness of voluntary movements, especially in the initiation of such movements as walking or rolling over in bed;
- Decreased facial expression, monotonous speech, and decreased eye **blinking**;
- A **shuffling gait** with poor arm swing and **stooped** posture;
- Unsteady balance;
- Difficulty rising from a sitting position;
- Continuous "pill-rolling" motion of the thumb and forefinger;
- Abnormal tone or stiffness in the trunk and **extremities**;
- Swallowing problems in later stages;
- Light headedness or fainting when standing (**orthostatic hypotension**).

Diagnosis

If you have at least two of these main signs, your doctor will want to find out if Parkinson's disease is the reason behind them:

- Tremor or shaking;
- Slow movement (called **bradykinesia**);
- Stiff or rigid arms, legs, or trunk;
- Balance problems or frequent falls.

Examination

If your doctor thinks you might have Parkinson's disease, they'll recommend that you see a specialist who works with nervous system issues, called a neurologist. Your neurologist will probably want to see how well your arms and legs move and check your muscle tone and balance. They may ask you to get out of a chair without using your arms for support, for example. They also may ask a few questions. Tell your doctor if you've noticed a change in your sense of smell or you have trouble with sleep, memory, or mood. Parkinson's disease can look different from person to person. Many people have some symptoms and not others.

Tests

Your doctor may want to start by testing your blood or doing a brain scan to rule out other conditions.

People who have Parkinson's disease don't make enough of a brain chemical called dopamine, which helps you move. If those first tests don't show a reason for your symptoms, your doctor may ask you to try a medication called **carbidopa-levodopa**, which your brain can turn into dopamine. If your symptoms get much better after you start the drug, your doctor probably will tell you that you have Parkinson's disease.

If the medication doesn't work for you and there's no other explanation for your issues, your doctor might suggest an imaging test called a DaTscan. This uses a small amount of a radioactive drug and a special scanner, called a single photon emission computed tomography (SPECT) scanner, to see how much dopamine is in your brain. This test can't tell you for sure that you have Parkinson's disease, but it can give your doctor more information to work with.

Treatment

If you have Parkinson's disease, you have a lot of choices for treatment. There's no cure, but medicine and sometimes surgery can help.

Your doctor may suggest you try one of these drugs:

Levodopa. It's a drug that doctors prescribe most often for Parkinson's. Levodopa may improve your symptoms because it is converted to dopamine in the brain.

Dopamine agonists. These are drugs that imitate the action of dopamine in your brain. Some examples are pramipexole, and rotigotine. You can take them alone or with L-dopa to treat the motor symptoms of Parkinson's disease.

COMT inhibitors. You take these drugs, such as entacapone (Comtan), opicapone (Ongentys) and tolcapone (Tasmar), along with levodopa. They add to the amount of time you get relief from symptoms by blocking the action of an enzyme that breaks down levodopa. Tolcapone is rarely prescribed by doctors, though, because it can cause liver damage.

MAO-B inhibitors. They also block the action of an enzyme that breaks down dopamine. You can take them alone early in Parkinson's disease or with other drugs as your disease moves to a later stage. MAO-B inhibitors include rasagiline (Azilect) and selegiline (Eldepryl, Zelapar). You usually take them alone because you can get side effects when you combine them with other drugs.

Other medications that doctors prescribe for Parkinson's include amantadine (Gocovri), apomorphine (Apokyn), and **anticholinergic** drugs. All can help control symptoms.

Other types of treatment for Parkinson's disease

Some people with Parkinson's have surgery called deep brain stimulation (DBS). In this procedure, doctors place a wire deep inside a specific spot in the brain, depending on the symptoms that need treatment. DBS can lead to dramatic improvements in many people.

Scientists are also exploring ways to place cells that make dopamine into the brain to help treat people with Parkinson's, instead of taking medicine. Some experts are trying to see if stem cells can be used for this, but research is still in an early stage.

Some treatments focus on the effects of the disorder, rather than the causes. Your doctor might refer you to a physical therapist to improve your balance and your ability to move. A physical therapist may also teach muscle-strengthening exercises to help you speak or swallow. It's important to keep up a daily exercise program and to stay socially active.

(1201 words)

◈ **Vocabulary**

Parkinson's disease ['pɑːkɪnsnz dɪziːz]［内科］帕金森病，震颤性麻痹

ganglion ['gæŋgliən] *n.* 神经节，神经中枢（复数 ganglia）

basal ganglia［解剖］基底神经节；［解剖］基底核

dopamine ['dəupəmiːn] *n.*［生化］多巴胺

（一种治脑神经病的药物）

acetylcholine [ˌæsɪtaɪl'kəuliːn] *n.*［有化］乙酰胆碱

neurotransmitter ['njuərəutrænzmɪtə] *n.* 神经传导物质

pesticide ['pestɪsaɪd] *n.* 杀虫剂

carbon monoxide [ˌkɑːbən mə'nɒksaɪd]

［无化］一氧化碳

manganese [ˈmæŋɡəniːz] n. ［化学］锰

parkinsonism [ˈpɑːkɪnsənɪzəm] n. 震颤麻痹；帕金森病

concussion [kənˈkʌʃn] n. 冲击，震荡；脑震荡

encephalitis [enˌsefəˈlaɪtɪs] n. ［内科］脑炎

neurological [ˌnjʊərəˈlɒdʒɪkl] adj. 神经病学的，神经学上的

blink [blɪŋk] vt. 眨眼，使……闪烁 vi. 眨眼，闪烁

shuffle [ˈʃʌf(ə)l] v. 拖着脚走

gait [ɡeɪt] n. 步法，步态

stoop [stuːp] vi. 弯腰；屈服；堕落 n. 弯腰，弯背；屈服

extremity [ɪkˈstreməti] n. 四肢，骨端；末端，极限

orthostatic hypotension ［内科］直立性低血压（= postural hypotension）

bradykinesia [breɪdaɪkɪˈniːzjə] n. 运动徐缓，动作迟缓

carbidopa-levodopa 帕金宁

levodopa [ˌliːvə(ʊ)ˈdəʊpə] n. ［药］左旋多巴（= L-dopa）

anticholinergic [ˌæntɪˌkɒlɪˈnɜːdʒɪk] adj. 反副交感神经生理作用的

◆ Exercises

Ⅰ. **Decide whether the following sentences are *True* or *False* according to the text.**

1. Parkinson's disease might be caused by the gradual degeneration of nerve cells in the portion of the midbrain that controls body movements.

2. Parkinson's disease usually begins between the ages of 50 and 65, and it is slightly more common in women than in men.

3. Parkinson's disease can't be cured, but medicine and sometimes surgery can help the symptoms.

4. The drug that doctors prescribe most for Parkinson's is the drug Levodopa, because it may improve your symptoms by converting to dopamine in the brain.

5. Treating Parkinson's disease is often done by your neurologist, without the help from wide variety of other specialists.

6. Genetics, viral infection, and brain tumor may cause Parkinson's disease, but hydrocephalus is not a risk factor.

7. Parkinsonism may not be present in persons with Alzheimer's disease, Wilson's disease, and Huntington's disease.

8. Orthostatic hypotension is not one of the symptoms of Parkinson's disease.

9. Tremor, stiffness and balance problems are not the main signs of Parkinson's disease.

10. Some people with Parkinson's have surgery called DBS, which a wire is put deep inside a specific spot in the brain.

II. Fill in the blanks with the proper form of words in the box.

dementia	psychosis	dopamine	encephalitis	concussion
hydrocephalus	ganglia	tomography	bradykinesia	agonist

1. _____ refers to obtain pictures of the interior of the body in medicine.

2. An _____ is a chemical that binds to a receptor and activates the receptor to produce a biological response.

3. _____ is abnormal slowing of voluntary movement, usually with a diminished range of movement.

4. He may have some kind of neurosis or _____ later in life.

5. There are pretty clear differences between signs of _____ and age-related memory loss.

6. _____ is an inflammation of the brain, usually caused by a direct viral infection or a hyper-sensitivity reaction to a virus or foreign protein.

7. _____ is a condition in which an accumulation of cerebrospinal fluid occurs within the brain.

8. He was taken to the hospital with a _____ caused by the car accident.

9. _____ is a neurotransmitter that plays several important roles in the brain and body.

10. A _____ is a group of neuron cell bodies in the peripheral nervous system.

III. Translation: translate the passage into Chinese.

Alzheimer's disease is the most common type of dementia. It is a progressive disease beginning with mild memory loss and possibly leading to loss of the ability to carry on a conversation and respond to the environment. Alzheimer's disease involves parts of the brain that control thought, memory, and language. It can seriously affect a person's ability to carry out daily activities. In 2020, as many as 5.8 million Americans were living with Alzheimer's disease. Younger people may get Alzheimer's disease, but it is less common. The number of people living with the disease doubles every 5 years beyond age 65. This number is projected to nearly 14 million people by 2060. Symptoms of the disease can first appear after age 60, and the risk increases with age. Scientists do not yet fully understand what causes Alzheimer's disease. There likely is not a single cause but rather several factors that can affect each person differently.

Alzheimer's disease is not a normal part of aging. Memory problems are typically one of the first warning signs of Alzheimer's disease and related dementias. In addition to memory problems, someone with symptoms of Alzheimer's disease may experience one or more of the following:

- Memory loss that disrupts daily life, such as getting lost in a familiar place or repeating questions.
  - Trouble handling money and paying bills.
  - Difficulty completing familiar tasks at home, at work or at leisure.
  - Decreased or poor judgment.
  - Misplacing things and being unable to retrace steps to find them.
  - Changes in mood, personality, or behavior.

Medical management can improve quality of life for individuals living with Alzheimer's disease and for their caregivers. There is currently no known cure for Alzheimer's disease. Treatment addresses several areas: helping people maintain brain health, managing behavioral symptoms and slowing or delaying symptoms of the disease.

(328 words)

Ⅳ. Give a presentation.

Dictate the causes, symptoms, treatments, etc. of Parkinson's Disease in English with 3—4 students. Try to use the formal expression, especially related medical terminology when you make your presentation.

Ⅴ. Describe the patient's past medical history in English.

根据下列内容,用英语描述既往病史。

1999 年冬天,病人上腹部中间出现间歇性钝痛,餐后缓解。此后每年冬天都会反复,有时伴有返酸或腹泻,但无呕吐。每次大约持续两到三周。病人自服胃舒平。在 2011 年,病人被诊断患十二指肠溃疡。

Text C

Epilepsy

Epilepsy is a central nervous system (neurological) disorder in which brain activity becomes abnormal, causing seizures or periods of unusual behavior, sensations, and sometimes loss of awareness.

Anyone can develop epilepsy. Epilepsy affects both males and females of all races, ethnic backgrounds and ages.

Seizure symptoms can vary widely. Some people with epilepsy simply stare blankly for a few seconds during a seizure, while others repeatedly twitch their arms or legs. Having a single seizure doesn't mean you have epilepsy. At least two unprovoked seizures are generally required for an epilepsy diagnosis.

Treatment with medications or sometimes surgery can control seizures for the majority of people with epilepsy. Some people require lifelong treatment to control seizures, but for others, the seizures eventually go away. Some children with epilepsy may outgrow the condition with age.

Symptoms

Because epilepsy is caused by abnormal activity in the brain, seizures can affect any process your brain coordinates. Seizure signs and symptoms may include:

- Temporary confusion;
- A staring spell;
- Uncontrollable jerking movements of the arms and legs;
- Loss of consciousness or awareness;
- **Psychic** symptoms such as fear, anxiety or *deja vu*.

Symptoms vary depending on the type of seizure. In most cases, a person with epilepsy will tend to have the same type of seizure each time, so the symptoms will be similar from episode to episode.

Causes

Epilepsy has no identifiable cause in about half the people with the condition. In the other half, the condition may be traced to various factors, including:

- Genetic influence. Some types of epilepsy run in families. In these cases, it's likely that there's a genetic influence.
- Head trauma. Head trauma as a result of a car accident or other traumatic injury can cause epilepsy.
- Brain conditions. Brain conditions that cause damage to the brain, such as brain tumors or strokes, can cause epilepsy. Stroke is a leading cause of epilepsy in adults older than age 35.
- Infectious diseases. Infectious diseases, such as **meningitis**, AIDS and viral encephalitis, can cause epilepsy.
- Prenatal injury. Before birth, babies are sensitive to brain damage that could be caused by several factors, such as an infection in the mother, poor nutrition or oxygen deficiencies. This brain damage can result in epilepsy or cerebral **palsy**.
- Developmental disorders. Epilepsy can sometimes be associated with developmental disorders, such as autism and **neurofibromatosis**.

Diagnosis

To diagnose your condition, your doctor will review your symptoms and medical history. Your doctor may order several tests to diagnose epilepsy and determine the cause of seizures. Your evaluation may include:

- A neurological exam. Your doctor may test your behavior, motor abilities, mental function and other areas to diagnose your condition and determine the type of epilepsy you may have.
- Blood tests. Your doctor may take a blood sample to check for signs of infections, genetic conditions or other conditions that may be associated with seizures.

Your doctor may also suggest tests to detect brain abnormalities, such as:

- **Electroencephalogram** (EEG). This is the most common test used to diagnose epilepsy. In this test, electrodes are attached to your scalp with a paste-like substance or cap. The electrodes record the electrical activity of your brain. If you have epilepsy, it's common to have changes in your normal pattern of brain waves, even when you're not having a seizure. Your doctor may monitor you on video when conducting an EEG while you're awake or asleep, to record any seizures you experience.
- High-density EEG. In a variation of an EEG test, your doctor may recommend high-density EEG, which spaces electrodes more closely than

conventional EEG—about a half a centimeter apart. High-density EEG may help your doctor more precisely determine which areas of your brain are affected by seizures.

• Computerized tomography (CT) scan. A CT scan uses X-rays to obtain cross-sectional images of your brain. CT scans can reveal abnormalities in your brain that might be causing your seizures, such as tumors, bleeding and **cysts**.

• Magnetic resonance imaging (MRI). An MRI uses powerful magnets and radio waves to create a detailed view of your brain. Your doctor may be able to detect lesions or abnormalities in your brain that could be causing your seizures.

• Functional MRI (fMRI). A functional MRI measures the changes in blood flow that occur when specific parts of your brain are working. Doctors may use an fMRI before surgery to identify the exact locations of critical functions, such as speech and movement, so that surgeons can avoid injuring those places while operating.

• **Positron emission tomography** (PET). PET scans use a small amount of low-dose radioactive material that's injected into a vein to help visualize active areas of the brain and detect abnormalities.

• Single-photon emission computerized tomography (SPECT). This type of test is used primarily if you've had an MRI and EEG that didn't pinpoint the location in your brain where the seizures are originating. A SPECT test uses a small amount of low-dose radioactive material that's injected into a vein to create a detailed, 3-D map of the blood flow activity in your brain during seizures.

• **Neuropsychological** tests. In these tests, doctors assess your thinking, memory and speech skills. The test results help doctors determine which areas of your brain are affected.

Along with your test results, your doctor may use a combination of analysis techniques to help pinpoint where in the brain seizures start:

• Statistical parametric mapping (SPM). SPM is a method of comparing areas of the brain that have increased metabolism during seizures to normal brains, which can give doctors an idea of where seizures begin.

• Curry analysis. Curry analysis is a technique that takes EEG data and projects it onto an MRI of the brain to show doctors where seizures are occurring.

• **Magnetoencephalography** (MEG). MEG measures the magnetic fields produced by brain activity to identify potential areas of seizure onset.

Accurate diagnosis of your seizure type and where seizures begin gives you the best chance for finding an effective treatment.

Treatment

Doctors generally begin by treating epilepsy with medication. If medications don't treat the condition, doctors may propose surgery or another type of treatment.

Medication

Most people with epilepsy can become seizure-free by taking one anti-seizure medication, which is also called anti-epileptic medication. Others may be able to decrease the frequency and intensity of their seizures by taking a combination of medications.

Many children with epilepsy who aren't experiencing epilepsy symptoms can eventually discontinue medications and live a seizure-free life. Many adults can discontinue medications after two or more years without seizures. Your doctor will advise you about the appropriate time to stop taking medications.

Finding the right medication and dosage can be complex. Your doctor will consider your condition, frequency of seizures, your age and other factors when choosing which medication to prescribe. He likely will first prescribe a single medication at a relatively low dosage and may increase the dosage gradually until your seizures are well-controlled.

Surgery

When medications fail to provide adequate control over seizures, surgery may be an option. With epilepsy surgery, a surgeon removes the area of your brain that's causing seizures. Doctors usually perform surgery when tests show that:

• Your seizures originate in a small, well-defined area of your brain.

• The area in your brain to be operated on doesn't interfere with vital functions such as speech, language, motor function, vision or hearing.

Although many people continue to need some medication to help prevent seizures after successful surgery, you may be able to take fewer drugs and reduce your dosages.

In a small number of cases, surgery for epilepsy can cause complications such as permanently altering your thinking (cognitive) abilities. Talk to your surgeon about his or her experience, success rates, and complication rates with the procedure you're considering.

(1302 words)

◆ Vocabulary

epilepsy ['epɪˌlepsi] *n.* 癫痫，癫痫症

psychic ['saɪkɪk] *adj.* 精神的，心灵的

deja vu [法语] 似曾相识的感觉，过分熟悉

meningitis [ˌmenɪn'dʒaɪtɪs] *n.* 脑膜炎

palsy ['pɔːlzi] *n.* 麻痹，麻痹状态　*vt.* 麻痹，使瘫痪

neurofibromatosis
　　[njʊərəʊ'faɪbrəʊmətəʊsɪs] *n.* 神经纤维瘤病

electroencephalogram
　　[ɪˌlektrəʊen'sefələˌgræm] *n.* ［内科］脑电图

cyst [sɪst] *n.* ［肿瘤］囊肿，［生物］包囊，膀胱

positron emission tomography ［生物物理］正电子放射断层造影术，正电子发射计算机断层显像

neuropsychological 神经心理学

magnetoencephalography
　　[mægniˌtəʊen'sefə'lɒgrəfi] *n.* 脑磁图描记术

Text D

Encephalitis

Encephalitis is inflammation of the brain. There are several causes, but the most common is a viral infection. Encephalitis often causes only mild flu-like signs and symptoms—such as a fever or headache—or no symptoms at all. Sometimes the flu-like symptoms are more severe. Encephalitis can also cause confused thinking, seizures, or problems with movement or with senses such as sight or hearing. In some cases, encephalitis can be life-threatening. Timely diagnosis and treatment are important because it's difficult to predict how encephalitis will affect each individual.

Symptoms

Most people with viral encephalitis have mild flu-like symptoms, such as:

- Headache;
- Fever;
- Aches in muscles or joints;
- Fatigue or weakness.

Sometimes the signs and symptoms are more severe, and might include:

- Confusion, agitation or hallucinations;
- Seizures;
- Loss of sensation or paralysis in certain areas of the face or body;
- Muscle weakness;
- Problems with speech or hearing;
- Loss of consciousness (including coma).

In infants and young children, signs and symptoms might also include:

- Bulging in the soft spots (**fontanels**) of an infant's skull;
- Nausea and vomiting;
- Body stiffness;
- Poor feeding or not waking for a feeding;
- Irritability.

Causes

The exact cause of encephalitis is often unknown. But when a cause is known, the most common is a viral infection. Bacterial infections and noninfectious inflammatory conditions also can cause encephalitis. There are two main types of encephalitis:

• Primary encephalitis. This condition occurs when a virus or other agent directly infects the brain. The infection may be concentrated in one area or widespread. A primary infection may be a reactivation of a virus that had been inactive after a previous illness.

• Secondary encephalitis. This condition results from a faulty immune system reaction to an infection elsewhere in the body. Instead of attacking only the cells causing the infection, the immune system also mistakenly attacks healthy cells in the brain. Also known as post-infection encephalitis, secondary encephalitis often occurs two to three weeks after the initial infection.

Common viral causes

The viruses that can cause encephalitis include:

• **Herpes simplex virus** (HSV). Both HSV type 1—associated with cold sores and fever blisters around your mouth—and HSV type 2—associated with genital herpes—can cause encephalitis. Encephalitis caused by HSV type 1 is rare but can result in significant brain damage or death.

• Other herpes viruses. These include the Epstein-Barr virus, which commonly causes infectious **mononucleosis**, and the **varicella-zoster** virus, which commonly causes **chickenpox** and **shingles**.

• **Enteroviruses**. These viruses include the **poliovirus** and the **coxsackievirus**, which usually cause an illness with flu-like symptoms, eye inflammation and abdominal pain.

• Mosquito-borne viruses. These viruses can cause infections such as West Nile, La Crosse, St. Louis, western equine and eastern **equine encephalitis**. Symptoms of an infection might appear within a few days to a couple of weeks after exposure to a mosquito-borne virus.

• **Tick**-borne viruses. The Powassan virus is carried by ticks and causes encephalitis in the Midwestern United States. Symptoms usually appear about a week after a bite from an infected tick.

• **Rabies** virus. Infection with the rabies virus, which is usually transmitted by a bite from an infected animal, causes a rapid progression to encephalitis once symptoms begin. Rabies is a rare cause of encephalitis in the United States.

• Childhood infections. Common childhood infections—such as **measles** (**rubeola**), **mumps** and German measles (**rubella**)—used to be fairly common causes of secondary encephalitis. These causes are now rare in the world due to the availability of vaccinations for these diseases.

Complications

The complications of encephalitis vary, depending on factors such as:

- Your age;
- The cause of your infection;
- The severity of your initial illness;
- The time from disease onset to treatment.

People with relatively mild illness usually recover within a few weeks with no long-term complications.

Complications of severe illness

Inflammation can injure the brain, possibly resulting in a coma or death. Other complications—varying greatly in severity—may persist for months or be permanent. These complications can include:

- Persistent fatigue;
- Weakness or lack of muscle coordination;
- Personality changes;
- Memory problems;
- Paralysis;
- Hearing or vision defects;
- Speech impairments.

Diagnosis

Your doctor will start with a thorough physical examination and medical history. Your doctor might then recommend:

• Brain imaging. MRI or CT images can reveal any swelling of the brain or another condition that might be causing your symptoms, such as a tumor.

• Spinal tap (lumbar puncture). A needle inserted into your lower back removes a small amount of **cerebrospinal** fluid (CSF), the protective fluid that surrounds the brain and spinal column. Changes in this fluid can indicate infection and inflammation in the brain. Sometimes samples of CSF can be tested to identify the virus or other infectious agent.

• Other lab tests. Samples of blood, urine or excretions from the back of the throat can be tested for viruses or other infectious agents.

• Electroencephalogram (EEG). Electrodes affixed to your scalp record the brain's electrical activity. Certain abnormal patterns may indicate a diagnosis of encephalitis.

• Brain biopsy. Rarely, a small sample of brain tissue might be removed for testing. A brain biopsy is usually done only if symptoms are worsening and treatments are having no effect.

Treatment

Treatment for mild encephalitis usually consists of:

• Bed rest;
• Plenty of fluids;
• Anti-inflammatory drugs—such as acetaminophen (Tylenol, others), ibuprofen (Advil, Motrin IB, others) and **naproxen** sodium (Aleve)—to relieve headaches and fevers.

Antiviral drugs
Encephalitis caused by certain viruses usually requires antiviral treatment.

Antiviral medications commonly used to treat encephalitis include:

• **Acyclovir** (Zovirax);
• Ganciclovir (Cytovene);
• **Foscarnet** (Foscavir).

Some viruses, such as insect-borne viruses, don't respond to these treatments. But because the specific virus may not be identified immediately or at all, doctors often recommend immediate treatment with acyclovir. Acyclovir can be effective against HSV, which can result in significant complications when not treated promptly. Antiviral medications are generally well tolerated. Rarely, side effects can include kidney damage.

Supportive care
People who are hospitalized with severe encephalitis might need:

• Breathing assistance, as well as careful monitoring of breathing and heart function;
• Intravenous fluids to ensure proper hydration and levels of essential minerals;
• Anti-inflammatory drugs, such as corticosteroids, to reduce swelling and pressure within the skull;
• Anticonvulsant medications, such as **phenytoin (Dilantin)**, to stop or prevent seizures.

Follow-up therapy

If you experience complications of encephalitis, you might need additional therapy, such as:

• Physical therapy to improve strength, flexibility, balance, motor coordination and mobility;

• Occupational therapy to develop everyday skills and to use adaptive products that help with everyday activities;

• Speech therapy to relearn muscle control and coordination to produce speech;

• Psychotherapy to learn coping strategies and new behavioral skills to improve mood disorders or address personality change.

(1160 words)

◆ **Vocabulary**

fontanel [ˌfɒntəˈnel] *n.* [中医][解剖] 囟门

herpes simplex virus [病毒] 单纯性疱疹病毒

mononucleosis [ˌmɒnəʊˌnjuːkliˈəʊsɪs] *n.* 单核细胞增多症

varicella [ˈværəˈselə] *n.* 水痘

zoster [ˈzɒstə(r)] *n.* 带状疱疹

chickenpox [ˈtʃɪkɪnˌpɒks] *n.* 水痘

shingles [ˈʃɪŋglz] *n.* [皮肤] 带状疱疹

enterovirus [ˌentərəʊˈvaɪərəs] *n.* [病毒] 肠道病毒

poliovirus [ˈpəʊliəʊˌvaɪərəs] *n.* 脊髓灰质炎病毒

coxsackievirus [kɒksækɪˈevaɪrəs] *n.* 柯萨奇病毒

equine encephalitis 马脑炎

tick [tɪk] *n.* 记号，滴答声；蜱

rabies [ˈreɪbiːz] *n.* 狂犬病，恐水症

measles [ˈmiːzlz] *n.* 麻疹

rubeola [ruˈbiːələ] *n.* 麻疹，风疹

mumps [mʌmps] *n.* 流行性腮腺炎；愠怒，生气

rubella [ruːˈbelə] *n.* 风疹

cerebrospinal [ˌserɪbrəʊˈspaɪnəl] *adj.* 脑脊髓的

naproxen [nəˈprɒksɪn] *n.* 萘普生，甲氧萘丙酸

acyclovir [eɪˈsaɪkləvɪə(r)] *n.* 阿昔洛韦（治疗疱疹的药物），无环鸟苷

foscarnet [fɒsˈkɑːnet] *n.* [药] 膦甲酸

phenytoin [ˈfenɪtɔɪn] *n.* [药] 苯妥英，二苯乙内酰脲

Dilantin [daɪˈlæntɪn] *n.* [药] 狄兰汀（可治癫痫）

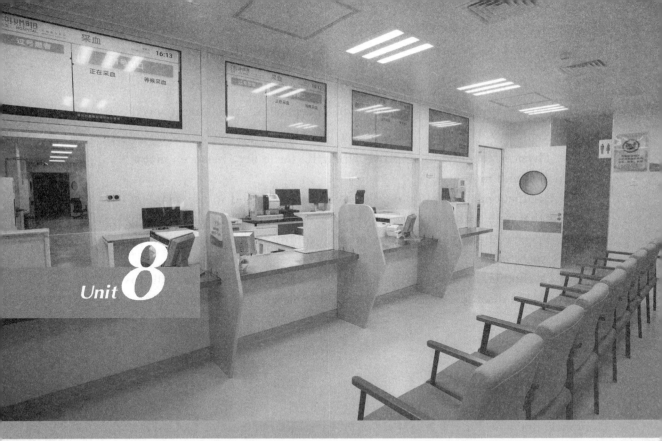

Unit 8

Some Common Diseases of the Skeletal System

✓参考答案
✓微课等资源

Text A

Fracture

A **fracture** is the medical term for a broken bone. Fractures are common; the average person has two during a lifetime. They occur when the physical force exerted on the bone is stronger than the bone itself.

Your risk of fracture depends, in part, on your age. Broken bones are very common in childhood, although children's fractures are generally less complicated than fractures in adults. As you age, your bones become more **brittle** and you are more likely to suffer fractures from falls that would not occur when you were young.

Types

There are many types of fractures, but the main categories are displaced, non-displaced, open, and closed. Displaced and non-displaced fractures refer to the **alignment** of the fractured bone.

In a **displaced fracture**, the bone snaps into two or more parts and moves so that the two ends are not lined up straight. If the bone is in many pieces, it is called a **comminuted fracture**. In a non-displaced fracture, the bone cracks either part or all of the way through, but does move and maintains its proper alignment.

A closed fracture is when the bone breaks but there is no puncture or open wound in the skin. An open fracture is one in which the bone breaks through the skin; it may then **recede** back into the wound and not be visible through the skin. This is an important difference from a closed fracture because with an open fracture there is a risk of a deep bone infection.

Because of the unique properties of their bones, there are some defined fracture subtypes that present only in children. For example:

- A greenstick fracture in which the bone is bent, but not broken all the way through.
- A **buckle** fracture results from compression of two bones driven into each other.
- A growth plate fracture at the joint that can result in shorter bone length.

These fracture subtypes can present in children and adults:

- A comminuted fracture is when the bone breaks into several pieces.
- A **transverse** fracture is when the fracture line is perpendicular to the shaft (long part) of the bone.
- An **oblique** fracture is when the break is on an angle through the bone.
- A pathologic fracture is caused by a disease that weakens the bone.
- A **stress fracture** is a hairline crack.

The severity of a fracture depends upon the fracture subtype and location. Serious fractures can have dangerous complications if not treated promptly; possible complications include damage to blood vessels or nerves and infection of the bone (**osteomyelitis**) or surrounding tissue. **Recuperation** time varies depending on the age and health of the patient and the type of fracture. A minor fracture in a child may heal within a few weeks; a serious fracture in an older person may take months to heal.

Symptoms

Signs and symptoms of a broken bone include:

- Swelling or bruising over a bone;
- Deformity of an arm or leg;
- Pain in the injured area that gets worse when the area is moved or pressure is applied;
- An inability to bear weight on the affected foot, ankle, or leg;
- Loss of function in the injured area;
- In open fractures, bone protruding from the skin.

Causes

Fractures are usually caused by a fall, blow, or other traumatic event.

Pathologic fractures are those caused by disease (such as cancer) that weakens the bones and can occur with little or no trauma. **Osteoporosis**, a disorder in which the bones thin and lose strength as they age, causes 1.5 million fractures each year in the U.S.—especially in the **hip**, wrist, and spine.

Diagnosis

Doctors can usually recognize most fractures by examining the injury and taking X-rays.

Sometimes an X-ray will not show a fracture. This is especially common with some wrist fractures, **hip** fractures (especially in older people), and stress fractures. In these situations, your doctor may perform other tests, such as a computed tomography (CT) scan, magnetic resonance imaging (MRI), or a bone scan.

In some cases, such as a possible wrist fracture with an initially normal X-ray, your doctor may apply a **splint** to immobilize the area and order a second X-ray 10 to 14 days later when healing can make the fracture visible.

Occasionally, even after the fracture diagnosis has been made, you may need other tests (such as a CT scan, MRI, or angiogram, a special X-ray of blood vessels) to determine whether other tissues around the bone have been damaged.

If your doctor suspects a skull fracture, they will probably skip plain X-rays altogether and proceed directly to a CT scan, which will diagnose the fracture and any more important related injuries or secondary injuries inside the skull, such as bleeding around the brain.

Treatment

A fracture often requires emergency treatment at a hospital. An example of a minor fracture that may not require emergency care is a fracture of the tip of a toe. If you think that bones may be broken in the back, neck, or hip or of bone is exposed, do not move the person; instead, call 911 (in the west) or 120 (in China) for help.

In other cases, you may call for assistance or transport the person to the emergency room. Before transporting the person, protect the injured area to avoid further damage. For broken arm or leg bones, put a splint (made of wood, plastic, metal, or another rigid material padded with **gauze**) against the area to prevent movement; loosely wrap the splint to the area using gauze. If there is bleeding, apply pressure to stop bleeding before splinting, then elevate the fracture.

Fractured bones must be set in their proper place and held there in order to heal properly. Setting a bone is called "reduction". Repositioning bone without surgery is "**closed reduction**". Most fractures in children are treated with closed reduction. Serious fractures may require open reduction—repositioning using surgery. In some cases, devices such as pins, plates, screws, rods, or glue are used to hold the fracture in place. Open fractures must also be cleaned thoroughly to avoid infection.

After setting, most fractures are immobilized with a cast, splint, or, occasionally, **traction** to reduce pain and help healing. In most cases, medication is limited to painkillers to reduce pain. In open fractures, antibiotics are administered to prevent infection. Rehabilitation begins as soon as possible, even if the bone is in a cast. This promotes blood flow, healing, maintenance of muscle tone, and helps prevent blood clots and stiffness.

After the cast or splint is removed, the area around the fracture usually is stiff for several weeks with swelling and bumps. In children, increased hair on the arms and legs due to irritation of the hair **follicles** from the cast can occur. With fractured legs, there may be a limp. Symptoms generally disappear within a few weeks.

If you have broken a bone, once the cast or splint is removed you should gradually begin using the area again. It may take another four to six weeks for the bone to regain past strength. Ask your doctor what activity type and intensity is safe for you, based on your fracture and overall health. Exercising in a swimming pool is generally a good way to rehabilitate bones.

Prevention

To help prevent fractures, follow general safety precautions, including:

• Always wear a seat belt when riding in a motor vehicle.

• Always wear the proper safety equipment (helmets and other protective pads) for recreational activities, such as bike riding, snowboarding, or contact sports.

• Keep walkways and stairs free of objects that could cause you to trip.

• If you have osteoporosis, engage in regular exercise to improve your strength and balance, which may help reduce falls.

• Discuss starting bone-building medications and supplements (like calcium and vitamin D) with your doctor.

• When you are on a ladder, avoid using the top step and be sure you have someone holding the ladder.

(1326 words)

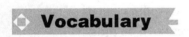 **Vocabulary**

fracture [ˈfræktʃə(r)] n. [外科] 骨折，破　　裂，断裂

brittle ['brɪtl] adj. 易碎的, 脆弱的; 易生气的

alignment [ə'laɪnmənt] n. 队列, 成直线; 校准

displaced fracture 移位的骨折

comminuted fracture [外科]粉碎性骨折

recede [rɪ'siːd] vi. 后退, 减弱 vt. 撤回

buckle ['bʌkl] n. 带扣, 搭钩 v. 扣住, 用搭扣装饰; 屈服, 退让; 使弯曲变形

transverse ['trænzvɜːs] adj. 横向的, 横断的

oblique [ə'bliːk] adj. 斜的; 不光明正大的

stress fracture [外科] 应力性骨折

osteomyelitis [ˌɒstɪəʊˌmaɪə'laɪtɪs] n. [外科]骨髓炎

recuperation [rɪˌkuːpə'reɪʃn] n. 恢复, 复原

osteoporosis [ˌɒstɪəʊpə'rəʊsɪs] n. [外科]骨质疏松症

hip [hɪp] n. 臀部

splint [splɪnt] n. 夹板, 薄木条; 薄金属片 vt. 用夹板固定

gauze [ɡɔːz] n. 纱布, 薄纱; 薄雾

closed reduction [外科]闭合复位术

traction ['trækʃn] n. 牵引; [机][车辆]牵引力

follicle ['fɒlɪkl] n. 小囊, 毛囊; 卵泡

◆ Exercises

Ⅰ. **Decide whether the following sentences are *True* or *False* according to the text.**

1. In a displaced fracture, the bone snaps into two or more parts and moves so that the two ends are not lined up straight.

2. There is a risk of a deep bone infection with open fracture, which makes an important difference from closed fracture.

3. Greenstick fracture, buckle fracture and growth plate fracture are present in children and adults.

4. Comminuted fracture, transverse fracture, oblique fracture and pathologic fracture are present only in adults.

5. Computed tomography (CT) scan, magnetic resonance imaging (MRI), or a bone scan will show a fracture, but sometimes an X-ray will not show a fracture.

6. If the cast or splint is removed from bone fracture, it may take four to six months for the bone to regain past strength.

7. Before transporting the person with bone fracture to hospital, put a splint against the area to prevent movement.

8. Greenstick fracture results from compression of two bones driven into each other.

9. Most fractures in children are treated with open reduction. Serious fractures may require closed reduction—repositioning using surgery.

10. A comminuted fracture is when the bone breaks into several pieces, while an oblique fracture is caused by a disease that weakens the bone.

Ⅱ. Fill in the blanks with the proper form of words in the box.

displace	osteomyelitis	oblique	deformity	comminuted
brittle	osteoporosis	angiogram	follicle	fracture

1. A _____ is one of the small hollows in the skin which hairs grow from.

2. _____ is a medical imaging technique used to visualize the inside, or lumen, of blood vessels and organs of the body.

3. The object of these movements is to prevent stiffness or _____ of joints.

4. _____ refers to a bone infection, almost always caused by a bacteria. Over time, the result can be destruction of the bone itself.

5. A(n) _____ fracture is when the break is on an angle through the bone.

6. A(n) _____ fracture is a fracture in which the bone is splintered or fragmented.

7. A(n) _____ fracture is the breakage in which the fragments are separated and are not in alignment.

8. _____ bone refers to bone that is abnormally fragile, as in osteogenesis imperfecta.

9. At least one-third of all women over ninety have sustained a hip _____.

10. _____ is a systemic skeletal disorder characterized by low bone mass, micro-architectural deterioration of bone tissue leading to bone fragility, and consequent increase in fracture risk.

Ⅲ. Translation: translate the passage into Chinese.

A hip fracture is a serious injury, with complications that can be life-threatening. The risk of hip fracture rises with age. Risk increases because bones tend to weaken with age (osteoporosis). Multiple medications, poor vision and balance problems also make older people more likely to fall—one of the most common causes of hip fracture. A hip fracture almost always requires surgical repair or replacement, followed by physical therapy. Taking steps to maintain bone density and avoid falls can help prevent a hip fracture.

Signs and symptoms of a hip fracture include: inability to get up from a fall or to walk, severe pain in your hip or groin, inability to put weight on your leg on the side of your injured hip, bruising and swelling in and around your hip area, shorter leg on the side of your injured hip, and outward turning of your leg on the side of your injured hip.

A severe impact—in a car crash, for example—can cause hip fractures in people of all ages. In older adults, a hip fracture is most often a result of a fall from a standing height. In people with very weak bones, a hip fracture can occur simply by standing on the leg.

The type of surgery you have generally depends on the where and how severe the fracture is, whether the broken bones aren't properly aligned (displaced), and your age and underlying health conditions. The options include:

• Internal repair using screws. Metal screws are inserted into the bone to hold it together while the fracture heals. Sometimes screws are attached to a metal plate that runs down the femur.

• Total hip replacement. Your upper femur and the socket in your pelvic bone are replaced with artificial parts (prostheses). Increasingly, studies show total hip replacement to be more cost-effective and associated with better long-term outcomes in healthy adults who live independently.

• Partial hip replacement. If the ends of the broken bone are displaced or damaged, your surgeon might remove the head and neck of the femur and install a metal replacement. Partial hip replacement might be recommended for adults who have other health conditions or cognitive impairment or who no longer live independently.

Your doctor might recommend partial or total hip replacement if the blood supply to the ball part of your hip joint was damaged during the fracture. That type of injury, which occurs most often in older people with femoral neck fractures, means the bone is less likely to heal properly.

(423 words)

Ⅳ. **Give a presentation.**

Dictate the causes, symptoms, treatments, etc. of Fracture in English with 3—4 students. Try to use the formal expression, especially related medical terminology when you make your presentation.

请根据下列内容,写一封会诊邀请信。

我院刚刚接收了一名病人,经初步诊断,疑似患有胰腺癌。但是有些迹象与诊断不符,而我们也无法做出其他的判断。邀请 Dr. Black 明天下午 2 点钟来我院一起讨论该病例。

Text B

Cervical Spondylosis

Cervical spondylosis is a general term for age-related wear and tear affecting the spinal disks in your neck. As the disks dehydrate and shrink, signs of **osteoarthritis** develop, including bony projections along the edges of bones (**bone spurs**).

Cervical spondylosis is very common and worsens with age. More than 85 percent of people older than age 60 are affected by cervical spondylosis.

Most people experience no symptoms from these problems. When symptoms do occur, nonsurgical treatments often are effective.

Symptoms

For most people, cervical spondylosis causes no symptoms. When symptoms do occur, they typically include pain and stiffness in the neck.

Sometimes, cervical spondylosis results in a narrowing of the space needed by the spinal cord and the nerve roots that pass through the spine to the rest of your body. If the spinal cord or nerve roots become **pinched**, you might experience:

- **Tingling**, numbness and weakness in your arms, hands, legs or feet;
- Lack of coordination and difficulty walking;
- Loss of bladder or bowel control.

Causes

As you age, the bones and cartilage that make up your backbone and neck gradually develop wear and tear. These changes can include:

- Dehydrated disks. Disks act like cushions between the **vertebrae** of your spine. By the age of 40, most people's spinal disks begin drying out and shrinking, which allows more bone-on-bone contact between the vertebrae.
- **Herniated disks**. Age also affects the exterior of your spinal disks. Cracks often appear, leading to bulging (herniated) disks—which sometimes can press on the spinal cord and nerve roots.
- Bone spurs. Disk degeneration often results in the spine producing extra amounts of bone in a misguided effort to strengthen the spine. These

bone spurs can sometimes pinch the spinal cord and nerve roots.

• Stiff ligaments. Ligaments are cords of tissue that connect bone to bone. Spinal ligaments can stiffen with age, making your neck less flexible.

Diagnosis

Your doctor will likely start with a physical exam that includes:

• Checking the range of motion in your neck;

• Testing your reflexes and muscle strength to find out if there's pressure on your spinal nerves or spinal cord;

• Watching you walk to see if spinal compression is affecting your gait.

Imaging tests

Imaging tests can provide detailed information to guide diagnosis and treatment. Your doctor might recommend:

• Neck X-ray. An X-ray can show abnormalities, such as bone spurs, that indicate cervical spondylosis. Neck X-ray can also rule out rare and more serious causes for neck pain and stiffness, such as tumors, infections or fractures.

• CT scan. A CT scan can provide more detailed imaging, particularly of bones.

• MRI. MRI can help pinpoint areas where nerves might be pinched.

• **Myelography**. A tracer dye is injected into the **spinal canal** to provide more detailed X-ray or CT imaging.

Nerve function tests

Your doctor might recommend tests to determine if nerve signals are traveling properly to your muscles. Nerve function tests include:

• **Electromyography**. This test measures the electrical activity in your nerves as they transmit messages to your muscles when the muscles are contracting and at rest.

• Nerve conduction study. Electrodes are attached to your skin above the nerve to be studied. A small shock is passed through the nerve to measure the strength and speed of nerve signals.

Treatment

Treatment for cervical spondylosis depends on the severity of your signs and symptoms. The goal of treatment is to relieve pain, help you maintain your usual activities as much as possible, and prevent permanent injury to the spinal cord and nerves.

Medications

If over-the-counter pain relievers aren't enough, your doctor might prescribe:

• Nonsteroidal anti-inflammatory drugs. While some types of NSAIDs are available over the counter, you may need prescription-strength versions to relieve the pain and inflammation associated with cervical spondylosis.

• Corticosteroids. A short course of oral **prednisone** might help ease pain. If your pain is severe, steroid injections may be helpful.

• Muscle relaxants. Certain drugs, such as **cyclobenzaprine**, can help relieve muscle spasms in the neck.

• Anti-seizure medications. Some epilepsy medications, such as **gabapentin** (Neurontin, Horizant) and **pregabalin** (Lyrica), can dull the pain of damaged nerves.

• Antidepressants. Certain antidepressant medications have been found to help ease neck pain from cervical spondylosis.

Therapy

A physical therapist can teach you exercises to help stretch and strengthen the muscles in your neck and shoulders. Some people with cervical spondylosis benefit from the use of traction, which can help provide more space within the spine if nerve roots are being pinched.

Surgery

If conservative treatment fails or if your neurological signs and symptoms—such as weakness in your arms or legs—worsen, you might need surgery to create more room for your spinal cord and nerve roots.

The surgery might involve:

• Removing a herniated disk or bone spurs;
• Removing part of a vertebra;
• Fusing a **segment** of the neck using bone graft and hardware.

Lifestyle and home remedies

Mild cervical spondylosis might respond to:

• Over-the-counter pain relievers. Ibuprofen (Advil, Motrin IB, others), naproxen sodium (Aleve) or acetaminophen (Tylenol, others) is often enough to control the pain associated with cervical spondylosis.

• Heat or ice. Applying heat or ice to your neck can ease sore neck muscles.

• Soft neck brace. The brace allows your neck muscles to rest.

However, a neck brace should be worn for only short periods of time because it can eventually weaken neck muscles.

- Regular exercise. Maintaining activity will help speed recovery, even if you have to temporarily modify some of your exercises because of neck pain. People who walk daily are less likely to experience neck and low back pain.

A person can ease the symptoms of cervical spondylosis with a few simple neck exercises.

Neck stretch

1. Keep your body straight.
2. Push your chin forward in a way that stretches the throat.
3. Softly tense the neck muscles.
4. Hold this for 5 seconds.
5. Return your head to its center position.
6. Push your head back with the chin held high, and hold for 5 seconds.
7. Carry out 5 repetitions (repeat 5 times).

Neck tilt

1. Tilt your head forward so that the chin touches the chest.
2. Softly tense the neck muscles.
3. Hold this for 5 seconds.
4. Return the head to a neutral position.
5. Carry out 5 repetitions.

Neck tilt (side-to-side)

1. Lean your head down towards either shoulder, leading with the ear.
2. Softly tense the neck muscles.
3. Hold this for 5 seconds.
4. Return your head to the center and repeat on the other shoulder.
5. Carry out 5 repetitions.

Neck turn

1. Turn your head to one side as far as it remains comfortable, being sure to keep your chin at a level height.
2. Tense your neck muscles for 5 seconds.
3. Return the head to a central position.
4. Repeat on the opposite side.
5. Repeat this exercise 5 times on each side.

These exercises can help to moderate the impact of the condition and alleviate pain or feelings of stiffness. However, they will not cure cervical spondylosis.

(1168 words)

◆ Vocabulary

cercical spondylosis 颈椎病

spondylosis [ˌspɒndɪˈləʊsɪs] *n.* 椎关节强硬

osteoarthritis [ˌɒstiəʊɑːˈθraɪtɪs] *n.* ［外科］骨关节炎

bone spur 骨刺

pinch [pɪntʃ] *v.* 捏，夹紧

tingle [ˈtɪŋgl] *v.* 感到刺痛，使激动

vertebra [ˈvɜːtɪbrə] *n.*[解剖]椎骨，脊椎（复数 vertebrae）

herniated disk ［外科］椎间盘突出

myelography [ˌmaɪəˈlɒgrəfi] *n.* 脊髓摄影术，脊髓造影术

spinal canal 椎管，脊管

electromyography [ɪˌlektrəʊmaɪˈɒgrəfi] *n.* ［物]肌电描记术，肌电图学

prednisone [ˈprednəˌsəʊn] *n.* ［药］泼尼松（肾上腺皮质激素）

cyclobenzaprine [ˌsaɪkləʊˈbenzəpriːn] *n.* 环苯扎林

gabapentin [gæbeɪˈpentɪn] *n.* 加巴喷丁

pregabalin [prɪgæˈbeɪlɪn] *n.* 普加巴林（一种新型抗癫痫药物），普瑞巴林

segment [ˈsegmənt] *n.* 部分，段，节

tilt [tɪlt] *n.* 倾斜　*v.* 倾斜，翘起

◆ Exercises

Ⅰ. **Decide whether the following sentences are *True* or *False* according to the text.**

1. As the spinal disks in your neck dehydrate and shrink, bone spurs can develop.

2. Cervical spondylosis worsens with age and older people are more easily affected by it.

3. Most people will experience symptoms of cervical spondylosis, such as pain in the neck.

4. Dehydrated disks mean people's spinal disks begin drying out and shrinking.

5. Sometimes herniated disks and bone spurs can pinch the spinal cord and nerve roots.

6. Neck X-ray and electromyography can help doctors to diagnose cervical spondylosis.

7. Medications, including corticosteroids can relieve pain from cervical spondylosis, but antidepressants are excluded.

8. Neck brace can be worn for long periods of time, and it can't weaken neck muscles.

9. Neck stretch, neck tilt and neck turn can ease the symptoms of cervical

spondylosis.

10. You should keep on exercising because exercises can cure cervical spondylosis.

II. Fill in the blanks with the proper form of words in the box.

spondylosis	spasm	cord	ligament	cervical
electromyography	spinal	tingle	osteoarthritis	herniate

1. _____ is chronic inflammation of the joints, esp. those that bear weight, with pain and stiffness.

2. Your _____ is the row of bones down your back.

3. A(n) _____ disk in the cervical region may cause arm pain and numbness.

4. _____ is a technique for recording the electrical activity of muscles and diagnosing the nerve and muscle disorders.

5. He suffered torn _____ in his knee while playing badminton.

6. Cervical _____ is a very common condition that usually occurs in the second half of life.

7. The cold made my ears _____ and I covered them with my hands.

8. The _____ is the entrance to the womb.

9. Your spinal _____ is a thick cord of nerves inside your spine which connects your brain to nerves in all parts of your body.

10. A muscular _____ in the coronary artery can cause a heart attack.

III. Translation: translate the passage into Chinese.

Top 10 Natural Home Remedies For Cervical Spondylosis Pain

Cervical spondylosis is a very popular age-related condition that affects your joints in the neck. It occurs because of wear and tear of the cartilage, bones and tissues of the cervical spine. There are several easy yet effective treatments to treat this problem. VKool.com will show you top 10 natural home remedies for cervical spondylosis pain.

1. Regular exercise

Lack of regular exercise is one of the major causes of cervical spondylosis. Hence, you can reduce stiffness and pain around your shoulders and neck by integrating regular physical exercise into your lifestyle.

2. Hot and cold compresses

Alternating cold and hot compresses on the affected area is one of the best home remedies for cervical spondylosis pain. Cold compresses will reduce inflammation and swelling while hot compresses will relax sore muscles and improve blood circulation as well.

3. Epsom salt bath

Taking an Epsom salt bath is one of the good home remedies for cervical spondylosis pain. The magnesium present in Epsom salt manages the PH levels in your body, in turn reducing stiffness, pain and inflammation in the shoulders and neck.

4. Garlic

Garlic is also considered as the effective home remedies for cervical spondylosis pain. Its analgesic and anti-inflammatory properties help treat swelling, pain and inflammation in your neck and surrounding areas.

5. Turmeric

Turmeric is one of the popular home remedies for cervical spondylosis pain thanks to its anti-inflammatory properties. Moreover, turmeric increases blood circulation that helps decrease muscle stiffness as well as pain.

6. Sesame seeds

One popular home remedy to cope with cervical spondylosis is using sesame seeds. They are rich in magnesium, manganese, calcium, copper, phosphorus, zinc and vitamins K and D, which are effective for your bones as well as overall health. Sesame seeds oil is also effective in decreasing neck pain.

7. Ginger

Ginger is also one of the other popular natural home remedies for cervical spondylosis pain. Ginger is high in anti-inflammatory properties. Thus, it helps decrease inflammation and pain in your neck and surrounding areas.

8. Apple cider vinegar

Being rich in alkalizing and anti-inflammatory properties, apple cider vinegar is also a great home remedy for cervical spondylosis pain. In addition, it can effectively soothe inflammation and pain in the neck area.

9. Cayenne pepper

One of the other effective home remedies for cervical spondylosis pain is cayenne pepper. Due to its anti-inflammatory as well as analgesic properties, it helps reduce inflammation and pain in the neck.

10. Indian lilac

Indian lilac contains pain-suppressing as well as anti-inflammatory properties that can alleviate inflammation, swelling and pain in the neck caused by cervical spondylosis.

(440 words)

IV. Give a presentation.

Dictate the causes, symptoms, treatments, etc. of Cervical Spondylosis in English with 3—4 students. Try to use the formal expression, especially related medical terminology when you make your presentation.

V. Write a treatment plan.

根据下列内容,用英语描述治疗方案。

1. 入院：口服抗生素,卧床休息,多喝水。当症状出现恶化,家庭治疗后症状并无缓解,病人就需要住院治疗。

2. 盘尼西林 400,000 u(肌注),一天两次(皮试后)：盘尼西林是治疗链球菌感染的常用药。

3. 链霉素 0.15 mg(肌注),一天两次：头孢类是治疗链球菌侵入性感染的重要抗生素。

4. 西地兰首剂 0.2 mg(肌注),然后每隔 6 小时 0.1 mg(肌注)两次。

Text C

Spinal Stenosis

Spinal stenosis is a narrowing of the spaces within your spine, which can put pressure on the nerves that travel through the spine. Spinal stenosis occurs most often in the lower back and the neck. Some people with spinal stenosis may not have symptoms. Others may experience pain, tingling, numbness and muscle weakness. Symptoms can worsen over time.

Spinal stenosis is most commonly caused by wear-and-tear changes in the spine related to osteoarthritis. In severe cases of spinal stenosis, doctors may recommend surgery to create additional space for the spinal cord or nerves.

Symptoms

Many people have evidence of spinal stenosis on an MRI or CT scan but may not have symptoms. When they do occur, they often start gradually and worsen over time. Symptoms vary depending on the location of the stenosis and which nerves are affected.

In the neck (cervical spine)
- Numbness or tingling in a hand, arm, foot or leg;
- Weakness in a hand, arm, foot or leg;
- Problems with walking and balance;
- Neck pain;
- In severe cases, bowel or bladder dysfunction (urinary urgency and incontinence).

In the lower back (lumbar spine)
- Numbness or tingling in a foot or leg;
- Weakness in a foot or leg;
- Pain or cramping in one or both legs when you stand for long periods of time or when you walk, which usually eases when you bend forward or sit;
- Back pain.

Causes

The backbone (spine) runs from your neck to your lower back. The bones of your spine form a spinal canal, which protects your spinal cord (nerves). Some people are born with a small spinal canal. But most spinal stenosis occurs when something happens to narrow the open space within the spine. Causes of spinal stenosis may include:

• Overgrowth of bone. Wear and tear damage from osteoarthritis on your spinal bones can prompt the formation of bone spurs, which can grow into the spinal canal. Paget's disease, a bone disease that usually affects adults, also can cause bone overgrowth in the spine.

• Herniated disks. The soft cushions that act as shock absorbers between your vertebrae tend to dry out with age. Cracks in a disk's exterior may allow some of the soft inner material to escape and press on the spinal cord or nerves.

• Thickened ligaments. The tough cords that help hold the bones of your spine together can become stiff and thickened over time. These thickened ligaments can bulge into the spinal canal.

• Tumors. Abnormal growths can form inside the spinal cord, within the membranes that cover the spinal cord or in the space between the spinal cord and vertebrae. These are uncommon and identifiable on spine imaging with an MRI or CT.

• Spinal injuries. Car accidents and other trauma can cause **dislocations** or fractures of one or more vertebrae. Displaced bone from a spinal fracture may damage the contents of the spinal canal. Swelling of nearby tissue immediately after back surgery also can put pressure on the spinal cord or nerves.

Diagnosis

To diagnose spinal stenosis, your doctor may ask you about signs and symptoms, discuss your medical history, and conduct a physical examination. He or she may order several imaging tests to help pinpoint the cause of your signs and symptoms.

Imaging tests may include:

• X-rays. An X-ray of your back can reveal bony changes, such as bone spurs that may be narrowing the space within the spinal canal. Each X-ray involves a small exposure to radiation.

• Magnetic resonance imaging (MRI). An MRI uses a powerful magnet and radio waves to produce cross-sectional images of your spine. The test can detect damage to your disks and ligaments, as well as the presence of tumors. Most important, it can show where the nerves in the spinal cord are being pressured.

• CT or CT **myelogram**. If you can't have an MRI, your doctor may recommend computerized tomography (CT), a test that combines X-ray images taken from many different angles to produce detailed, cross-sectional images of your body. In a CT myelogram, the CT scan is conducted after a contrast dye is injected. The dye outlines the spinal cord and nerves, and it can reveal herniated disks, bone spurs and tumors.

Treatment

Treatment for spinal stenosis depends on the location of the stenosis and the severity of your signs and symptoms. Talk to your doctor about the treatment that's best for your situation. If your symptoms are mild or you aren't experiencing any, your doctor may monitor your condition with regular follow-up appointments. He or she may offer some self-care tips that you can do at home. If these don't help, he or she may recommend medications or physical therapy. Surgery may be an option if other treatments haven't helped.

Medications

Your doctor may prescribe:

• Pain relievers. Pain medications such as ibuprofen (Advil, Motrin IB, others), naproxen (Aleve, others) and acetaminophen(Tylenol, others) may be used temporarily to ease the discomfort of spinal stenosis. They are typically recommended for a short time only, as there's little evidence of benefit from long-term use.

• Antidepressants. Nightly doses of tricyclic antidepressants, such as amitriptyline, can help ease chronic pain.

• Anti-seizure drugs. Some anti-seizure drugs, such as gabapentin (Neurontin) and pregabalin (Lyrica), are used to reduce pain caused by damaged nerves.

• **Opioids**. Drugs that contain **codeine**-related drugs such as **oxycodone** (Oxycontin, Roxicodone) and **hydrocodone** (Norco, Vicodin) may be useful for short-term pain relief. Opioids may also be considered cautiously for long-term treatment. But they carry the risk of serious side effects, including becoming habit forming.

Physical therapy

It's common for people who have spinal stenosis to become less active, in an effort to reduce pain. But that can lead to muscle weakness, which can result in more pain. A physical therapist can teach you exercises that may help:

- Build up your strength and endurance;
- Maintain the flexibility and stability of your spine;
- Improve your balance.

Steroid injections

Your nerve roots may become irritated and swollen at the spots where they are being pinched. While injecting a steroid medication (corticosteroid) into the space around **impingement** won't fix the stenosis, it can help reduce the inflammation and relieve some of the pain.

Steroid injections don't work for everyone. And repeated steroid injections can weaken nearby bones and connective tissue, so you can only get these injections a few times a year.

Decompression procedure

With this procedure, needle-like instruments are used to remove a portion of a thickened ligament in the back of the spinal column to increase spinal canal space and remove nerve root impingement. Only patients with lumbar spinal stenosis and a thickened ligament are eligible for this type of **decompression**.

The procedure is called **percutaneous image-guided** lumbar decompression (PILD). Because PILD is performed without general anesthesia, it may be an option for some people with high surgical risks from other medical problems.

Surgery

Surgery may be considered if other treatments haven't helped or if you're disabled by your symptoms. The goals of surgery include relieving the pressure on your spinal cord or nerve roots by creating more space within the spinal canal. Surgery to decompress the area of stenosis is the most definitive way to try to resolve symptoms of spinal stenosis.

Research shows that spine surgeries result in fewer complications when done by highly experienced surgeons. Examples of surgical procedures to treat spinal stenosis include:

- **Laminectomy**;
- **Laminotomy**;
- **Laminoplasty**;
- Minimally invasive surgery.

（1243 words）

◇ **Vocabulary**

spinal stenosis 椎管狭窄症

dislocation [ˌdɪsləˈkeɪʃn] n. 转位；混乱，[医] 脱臼

myelogram [maɪˈeləˌɡræm] n. 脊髓 X 光像，脊髓造影

opioid [əʊˈpiːɔɪd] n. 类鸦片 adj. 类鸦片的

codeine [ˈkəʊdiːn] n. 可待因（用鸦片制成的止痛镇咳药）

oxycodone [ˌɒksɪˈkəʊdəʊn] n. 氧可酮，羟考酮

hydrocodone [ˌhaɪdrəˈkəʊdəʊn] n. 氢可酮，二氢可待因酮

impingement [ɪmˈpɪndʒmənt] n. 冲击，影响；侵犯

decompression [ˌdiːkəmˈpreʃn] n. 解压，降压

percutaneous [ˌpɜːkjuːˈteɪniəs] adj. 经皮的，经由皮肤的

image-guided [ˈɪmɪdʒ ˈɡaɪdɪd] adj. 影像导航

laminectomy [ˌlæmɪˈnektəmi] n. ［外科］椎板切除术

laminotomy [ˌlæmaɪnəʊtəmi] n. ［外科］椎板切开术

laminoplasty [ˌlæmɪnɒpˈlæsti] n. ［外科］椎板成形术

Text D

Tenosynovitis

Tendinitis is when something—injury, illness, repeated motion—inflames one of your **tendons**, the cords of tissue that hold muscle to bone. When it also irritates the sleeve of tissue, or **sheath**, around the tendon, you have **tenosynovitis**.

Symptoms

The inflamed tendon may be painful and swollen. You may notice it more when you use it, especially if a repeated motion like swinging a hammer or a tennis **racquet** caused it.

When the tendon sheath gets swollen, fluid can build up and make your symptoms worse. You may feel swelling and in some cases see it, too. The area can get so tender that it hurts even to touch it.

It might happen anywhere you have muscles and tendons, but it's more likely in your:

- Shoulder;
- Upper arm;
- Forearm (**biceps**);
- Hands and fingers;
- Knee;
- Achilles (thick, **ropey** tissue that runs from **calf muscle** to heel).

If you have these symptoms in your thumb, then you probably have a specific type called De Quervain's tenosynovitis. It results from an inflamed tendon at the base of your thumb. You might feel:

- Pain along the thumb-side of the wrist;
- A catching or clicking when you use it;
- Your symptoms typically worsen when you try to squeeze or grab something or turn your wrist.

And you're more likely to get it when you're pregnant, though doctors aren't sure why.

Causes and risk factors

It isn't always clear what causes tenosynovitis (or tendinitis), though it usually starts in middle age. Repeated motions like jumping, throwing, or running might be to blame, or it might happen if you do something sudden like lifting an unusually heavy load. New movements, especially over your head, like painting the ceiling, also could play a role.

Arthritis and inflammatory diseases that wear down your joints may cause problems in surrounding tendons and tissues. This can sometimes lead to the long-term, or chronic, form of tenosynovitis. Serious cases can form cysts that tear or break tendons, change the shape of your hand, and make it hard to use.

Certain medicines like **fluoroquinolone** antibiotics (Cipro, Noroxin) and statins, which treat high cholesterol, also might raise your risk for tendon damage that leads to tenosynovitis.

Diagnosis

The doctor can usually diagnose you from your symptoms and a physical exam. They might push on affected areas or ask you to make specific motions and see if they hurt. Let them know how the area feels. Does it tingle? Burn? Does it get better when you rest? Be sure to tell them about any new increase in work or exercise patterns. If all this isn't enough to diagnose you, the doctor might take pictures of the area with an MRI or ultrasound machine to confirm or to rule out other causes.

Treatment

Rest is usually the first treatment. The quicker you start, the better it will work. Where possible, try to stop the things that cause your symptoms. You might even need a splint or brace to keep that part of your body from moving.

When it flares up, ice the inflamed area for 20 minutes at a time. Heat might be more useful for chronic tendinitis. Talk to your doctor if you're unsure.

Over-the-counter medications like nonsteroidal anti-inflammatory drugs (NSAIDs) can also help. Your doctor might suggest larger than standard doses depending on your level of pain and swelling or if you have conditions like **rheumatoid** arthritis. In some cases, they might inject a corticosteroid to reduce inflammation.

Once swelling and pain are down, you should start to slowly and gently increase your range of motion. If your tenosynovitis is severe, your doctor or physical therapist might give you a set of exercises to help with this. You may need to do them several times a day.

In rare cases, you might need surgery to repair a tendon or remove hard bits of calcium that can build up and cause tendon problems.

Tips

Tenosynovitis typically starts with tendinitis. Though it isn't always clear what causes either one, there are some things you can do that might lower your risk.

Take breaks. Try not to stay in the same position for too long. For example, if work keeps you still for hours on end, take breaks and move around every 30 minutes or so if you can. Don't do the same thing over and over without a break. Whether it's typing, throwing a baseball, or playing piano scales, mix up your movements to stay balanced and to give your body a chance to rest.

Learn how to lift. Take care when you lift things. Use a firm but not overly tight grip when it's unusually heavy, and avoid lifting with just one arm or only one side of your body.

Move the right way. Learn the right way to do the physical movements for all your sports and activities. Whether you lift weights, shoot free throws, or play the cello, there are proper techniques that can prevent injury. Trainers, teachers, coaches, and physical therapists can help you learn proper form. If you notice that some movement causes pain, stop and ask questions.

Living with tenosynovitis

It's important to rest as soon as you notice symptoms. If you don't, you could rupture a tendon or its sheath, which can be hard to repair. If your symptoms are very painful, won't go away, or stop you from living your life normally for more than a few days, see your doctor. They might notice an underlying condition that you can treat. They'll give you the right mix of rest, medication, and physical therapy to get you on the road to recovery.

(975 words)

tendinitis [ˌtendəˈnaɪtɪs] *n.* 腱炎

tendon [ˈtendən] *n.* 腱

sheath [ʃiːθ] *n.* 鞘

tenosynovitis [tenəʊsɪnəˈvaɪtɪs] *n.* 腱鞘炎

racquet [ˈrækɪt] *n.* 球拍

bicep [ˈbaɪseps] *n.* 二头肌（上臂前侧的主要肌肉）

ropey [ˈrəʊpi] *adj.* （非正式）破旧的，劣质的；不舒服的

calf muscle [医] 腓肠肌

fluoroquinolone [fluərəʊkwaɪnəˈləʊn] *n.* [医] 氟喹诺酮

rheumatoid [ˈruːmətɔɪd] *adj.* 类风湿病的

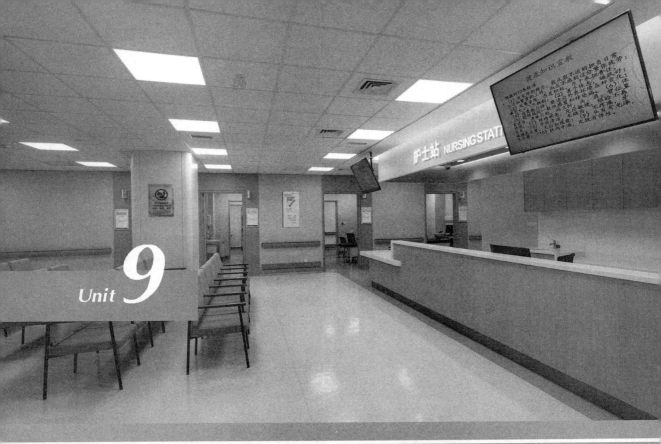

Unit *9*

Some Common Diseases of the Muscular System

✓参考答案
✓微课等资源

Text A

ACL Injury

An **ACL injury** is a tear or sprain of the **anterior cruciate** ligament (ACL)—one of the strong bands of tissue that help connect your **thigh** bone (**femur**) to your **shinbone** (**tibia**). ACL injuries most commonly occur during sports that involve sudden stops or changes in direction, jumping and landing—such as soccer, basketball, football and downhill skiing. Many people hear a pop or feel a "**popping**" sensation in the knee when an ACL injury occurs. Your knee may swell, feel unstable and become too painful to bear weight.

Depending on the severity of your ACL injury, treatment may include rest and rehabilitation exercises to help you regain strength and stability, or surgery to replace the torn ligament followed by rehabilitation. A proper training program may help reduce the risk of an ACL injury.

Symptoms

Signs and symptoms of an ACL injury usually include:

- A loud pop or a "popping" sensation in the knee;
- Severe pain and inability to continue activity;
- Rapid swelling;
- Loss of range of motion;
- A feeling of instability or "giving way" with weight bearing.

Causes

Ligaments are strong bands of tissue that connect one bone to another. The ACL, one of two ligaments that cross in the middle of the knee, connects your thigh bone to your shinbone and helps stabilize your **knee joint**. ACL injuries often happen during sports and fitness activities that can put stress on the knee:

- Suddenly slowing down and changing direction (cutting);
- **Pivoting** with your foot firmly planted;
- Landing awkwardly from a jump;
- Stopping suddenly;

- Receiving a direct blow to the knee or having a collision, such as a football tackle.

When the ligament is damaged, there is usually a partial or complete tear of the tissue. A mild injury may stretch the ligament but leave it intact.

Risk factors

There are a number of factors that increase your risk of an ACL injury, including:

- Being female—possibly due to differences in **anatomy**, muscle strength and hormonal influences;
- Participating in certain sports, such as soccer, football, basketball, gymnastics and downhill skiing;
- Poor conditioning;
- Using faulty movement patterns, such as moving the knees inward during a **squat**;
- Wearing footwear that doesn't fit properly;
- Using poorly maintained sports equipment, such as ski bindings that aren't adjusted properly;
- Playing on artificial **turf**.

Complications

People who experience an ACL injury have a higher risk of developing osteoarthritis in the knee. Arthritis may occur even if you have surgery to reconstruct the ligament.

Multiple factors likely influence the risk of arthritis, such as the severity of the original injury, the presence of related injuries in the knee joint or the level of activity after treatment.

Diagnosis

During the physical exam, your doctor will check your knee for swelling and tenderness—comparing your injured knee to your uninjured knee. He or she may also move your knee into a variety of positions to assess range of motion and overall function of the joint.

Often the diagnosis can be made on the basis of the physical exam alone, but you may need tests to rule out other causes and to determine the severity of the injury. These tests may include:

• X-rays. X-rays may be needed to rule out a bone fracture. However, X-rays don't show soft tissues, such as ligaments and tendons.

• Magnetic resonance imaging (MRI). An MRI uses radio waves and a strong magnetic field to create images of both hard and soft tissues in your body. An MRI can show the extent of an ACL injury and signs of damage to other tissues in the knee, including the cartilage.

• Ultrasound. Using sound waves to visualize internal structures, ultrasound may be used to check for injuries in the ligaments, tendons and muscles of the knee.

Treatment

Prompt first-aid care can reduce pain and swelling immediately after an injury to your knee. Follow the R.I.C.E. model of self-care at home:

• Rest. General rest is necessary for healing and limits weight bearing on your knee.

• Ice. When you're awake, try to ice your knee at least every two hours for 20 minutes at a time.

• **Compression**. Wrap an elastic bandage or compression wrap around your knee.

• Elevation. Lie down with your knee propped up on pillows.

Rehabilitation

Medical treatment for an ACL injury begins with several weeks of rehabilitative therapy. A physical therapist will teach you exercises that you will perform either with continued supervision or at home. You may also wear a brace to stabilize your knee and use **crutches** for a while to avoid putting weight on your knee.

The goal of rehabilitation is to reduce pain and swelling, restore your knee's full range of motion, and strengthen muscles. This course of physical therapy may successfully treat an ACL injury for individuals who are relatively inactive, engage in moderate exercise and recreational activities, or play sports that put less stress on the knees.

Surgery

Your doctor may recommend surgery if:

• You're an athlete and want to continue in your sport, especially if the sport involves jumping, cutting or pivoting;

• More than one ligament or the fibrous cartilage in your knee also is injured;

- The injury is causing your knee to buckle during everyday activities.

During ACL reconstruction, the surgeon removes the damaged ligament and replaces it with a segment of tendon—tissue similar to a ligament that connects muscle to bone. This replacement tissue is called a graft.

Your surgeon will use a piece of tendon from another part of your knee or a tendon from a **deceased** donor.

After surgery you'll resume another course of rehabilitative therapy. Successful ACL reconstruction paired with rigorous rehabilitation can usually restore stability and function to your knee.

There's no set time frame for athletes to return to play. Recent research indicates that up to one-third of athletes sustain another tear in the same or opposite knee within two years. A longer recovery period may reduce the risk of re-injury.

In general, it takes as long as a year or more before athletes can safely return to play. Doctors and physical therapists will perform tests to gauge your knee's stability, strength, function and readiness to return to sports activities at various intervals during your rehabilitation. It's important to ensure that strength, stability and movement patterns are **optimized** before you return to an activity with a risk of ACL injury.

(1079 words)

◆ **Vocabulary**

ACL injury 膝关节前交叉韧带损伤

anterior [æn'tɪəriə] *adj.*(空间上)位于前部的,前面的,向前的

cruciate ['kruːʃɪət] *adj.* 十字状的,十字形的,交叉的

thigh [θaɪ] *n.* 大腿,股

femur ['fiːmə(r)] *n.* [解剖] 股骨,大腿骨

shinbone ['ʃɪnˌbəʊn] *n.* 胫骨

tibia ['tɪbɪə] *n.* 胫骨,[昆] 胫节(昆虫)

popping ['pɒpɪŋ] *adj.* 间歇的,凸出的 *n.* 突然跳出

knee joint 膝关节

pivot ['pɪvət] *v.* 把……置于枢轴上,在枢轴上转动 *n.* 枢轴

anatomy [ə'nætəmi] *n.* 解剖,解剖学,剖析

squat [skwɒt] *v.* 蹲坐,蹲举

turf [tɜːf] *n.* 草皮,泥炭;跑马场

compression [kəm'preʃn] *n.* 压缩,浓缩;压榨,压迫

crutch [krʌtʃ] *n.* 拐杖,支柱,依靠 *vt.* 用拐杖支撑,支持

deceased [dɪ'siːst] *adj.* 已故的 *n.* 死者

optimize ['ɒptɪmaɪz] *vt.* 使最优化,使完善 *vi.* 优化;持乐观态度

⬥ Exercises

Ⅰ. **Decide whether the following sentences are *True* or *False* according to the text.**

1. ACL is one of the strong bands of tissue that help connect your femur to phalanx.

2. ACL injuries most commonly occur during sports and you may feel so unstable and painful that your knee can't bear weight.

3. Rehabilitation exercises or surgery can treat ACL injury.

4. Rapid swelling is one of the symptoms of ACL injury, but loss of range of motion is not.

5. Tendon is the strong bands of tissue that connect one bone to another.

6. An ACL injury patient does not have a higher risk of developing osteoarthritis.

7. X-rays, MRI as well as ultrasound are the test ways to diagnose ACL injury.

8. Icing your knee is a way to treat ACL injury at home by yourself.

9. During ACL injury, if more than one ligament or the fibrous cartilage in your knee also is injured, the doctor may recommend surgery.

10. Successful ACL reconstruction alone can usually restore stability and function to your knee.

Ⅱ. **Fill in the blanks with the proper form of words in the box.**

jaw	ligament	anterior	graft	cartilage
femur	rehabilitation	hipbone	shinbone	patella

1. _____ is the longest and thickest bone of the human skeleton.

2. _____ is the inner and thicker of the two bones of the human leg between the knee and ankle.

3. After the surgery, he would need months of patient _____ to learn to use his new thumb.

4. As the tough elastic tissue, _____ serves as a supporting framework for softer tissues.

5. _____ refers to a tissue or organ transplanted from a donor to a recipient. In some cases the patient can be both donor and recipient.

6. The patient was referred to our clinic due to suspected _____ encephalocele.

7. The most common cause of acute traumatic hemarthrosis of the knee is an anterior cruciate _____ tear.

8. _____ refers to large flaring bone forming one half of the pelvis.

9. _____ refers to a small flat triangular bone in front of the knee that

protects the knee joint.

10. _____ refers to either of the bone structures containing the teeth.

Ⅲ. **Translation: translate the passage into Chinese.**

The term "myositis" refers to a general inflammation or swelling of the muscle. Many people have experienced sore muscles after vigorous exercise, a condition that is temporary and improves with rest. Other conditions that can cause muscle weakness and pain include infection, muscle injury from medications, inherited diseases, electrolyte imbalances, and thyroid disease.

More often, however, the term myositis is used to refer to a disease involving chronic inflammation of the muscles, often occurring together with other symptoms. This condition is also known as idiopathic inflammatory myopathy (IIM). The disease is highly variable and has been classified into a number of forms, including:

- Dermatomyositis (DM);
- Polymyositis (PM);
- Necrotizing myopathy (NM);
- Sporadic inclusion body myositis (SIBM);
- Juvenile forms of myositis (JM).

Inflammatory myopathies are autoimmune diseases, meaning the body's immune system, which normally fights infections and viruses, is misdirected and begins to attack the body's own normal, healthy tissue. Inflammatory myopathies are rare diseases. All forms combined affect an estimated 50,000 to 75,000 people in the United States. While it is still unclear what causes myositis, some scientists believe certain individuals have a genetic predisposition to develop an autoimmune disease, which is triggered by an environmental exposure to some triggers, such as infection, virus, toxin, or sunlight.

Symptoms of weakness, swelling, and muscle damage often appear gradually. Long before patients are diagnosed, they may have trouble getting up from a chair, climbing stairs, or grasping objects with their hands. Patients may fall, find it difficult to reach their arms up, have difficulty swallowing, or other symptoms. In addition to these symptoms, it's common for patients to experience other complications.

Myositis is often difficult to diagnose, because many physicians are unfamiliar with the disease and its symptoms. A typical diagnosis process for myositis patients begins with a medical history and physical examination. It may also include blood tests, muscle and skin biopsies, and a variety of other diagnostic tests.

Myositis is a rare disease, so it is also difficult to conduct adequate research to test new treatments. There is a lot of confusion among the medical community over how to effectively manage patients with myositis. Nevertheless, myositis is a serious illness that, in most cases, needs to be treated aggressively. With inadequate or no treatment, myositis can cause significant disability and even death. There is no cure for any of the forms of myositis.

(405 words)

Ⅳ. Give a presentation.

Dictate the causes, symptoms, treatments, etc. of ACL Injury in English with 3—4 students. Try to use the formal expression, especially related medical terminology when you make your presentation.

Ⅴ. Write a cover letter for contribution.

根据下列内容,写一封投稿信。

附件是研究论文《低龄儿童的阑尾包块》,请您审阅。全体作者已经阅读并同意该版本。该论文的任何部分均未在其他刊物出版或投稿,提交的文稿不存在任何利益冲突。期望早日收到评审意见。

Text B

Muscle Atrophy

The term **muscle atrophy** refers to the loss of muscle tissue. **Atrophied** muscles appear smaller than normal. Lack of physical activity due to an injury or illness, poor nutrition, genetics, and certain medical conditions can all contribute to muscle atrophy.

Muscle atrophy can occur after long periods of inactivity. If a muscle does not get any use, the body will eventually break it down to conserve energy.

Muscle atrophy that develops due to inactivity can occur if a person remains immobile while they recover from an illness or injury. Getting regular exercise and trying physical therapy may reverse this form of muscle atrophy.

People can treat muscle atrophy by making certain lifestyle changes, trying physical therapy, or undergoing surgery.

In this article, we look at some other causes, symptoms, and treatments of muscle atrophy.

Causes

Many factors can cause muscle atrophy, including:

Poor nutrition

Poor nutrition can give rise to numerous health conditions, including muscle atrophy.

Specifically, the International Osteoporosis Foundation warn that diets low in **lean** protein, fruits, and vegetables can lead to reductions in muscle mass.

Malnutrition-related muscle atrophy may develop as a result of medical conditions that impair the body's ability to absorb nutrients, such as:

- **irritable bowel syndrome**;
- **celiac** disease;
- cancer.

Cachexia is a complex metabolic condition that causes extreme weight loss and muscle atrophy. Cachexia can develop as a symptom of another underlying condition, such as cancer, HIV, or **multiple sclerosis** (MS). People who have cachexia may experience a significant loss of appetite or unintentional weight loss despite consuming a large number of calories.

Age

As a person gets older, their body produces fewer proteins that promote muscle growth. This reduction of available protein causes the muscle cells to shrink, resulting in a condition called **sarcopenia**.

According to a report, sarcopenia affects up to a third of people ages 60 and above. In addition to reduced muscle mass, sarcopenia can cause the following symptoms:

- weakness or **frailty**;
- poor balance;
- difficulty moving;
- lower endurance.

A loss of muscle mass may be an inevitable result of the natural aging process. However, it can increase the risk of injuries and negatively impact a person's overall quality of life.

Genetics

Spinal muscular atrophy (SMA) is a genetic disorder that causes a loss of motor nerve cells and muscle atrophy.

There are several different types of SMA that fall into the following categories:

- SMA linked to **chromosome** 5

These types of SMA occur due to a **mutation** in the SMN1 genes on chromosome 5. The mutations lead to a deficiency of the survival motor neuron protein. SMA typically develops in childhood but can develop at any point in life.

- SMA not linked to chromosome 5

Muscular **dystrophy** refers to a group of progressive conditions that cause loss of muscle mass and weakness. Muscular dystrophy occurs when one of the genes involved in protein production mutates. A person can inherit genetic mutations, but many occur naturally as the embryo develops.

Medical conditions

Diseases and chronic conditions that can contribute to muscle atrophy include:

- **Amyotrophic lateral sclerosis** (ALS): Also called Lou Gehrig's disease, ALS includes several types that damage the motor nerve cells that control the muscles.
- **MS**: This chronic condition occurs when the body's immune system attacks the central nervous system, causing harmful inflammation in the nerve fibers.
- **Arthritis**: Arthritis refers to inflammation of the joints that causes pain and stiffness. Arthritis can severely limit a person's mobility, which could lead to muscle disuse and atrophy.
- **Myositis**: The term myositis refers to inflammation of the muscles. This condition causes muscle weakness and pain. People can develop myositis after a viral infection or as a side effect of an autoimmune condition.
- **Polio**: This infectious disease attacks the nervous system. It causes flu-like symptoms and can result in permanent paralysis.

Neurological problems

An injury or condition can damage the nerves that control the muscles, resulting in a condition called **neurogenic** muscle atrophy.

When this develops, the muscles stop contracting because they no longer receive signals from the nerve.

Symptoms

The symptoms of muscle atrophy vary widely depending on the cause and severity of muscle loss. In addition to reduced muscle mass, symptoms of muscle atrophy include:

- having one arm or leg that is noticeably smaller than the others;
- experiencing weakness in one limb or generally;
- having difficulty balancing;
- remaining inactive for an extended period.

Treatment

Treatment for muscle atrophy varies depending on the degree of muscle loss and the presence of any underlying medical conditions. Treating the underlying condition causing the muscle atrophy may help slow down the progression of the muscle loss. Treatment for muscle atrophy includes:

Physical therapy

Physical therapy involves performing specific stretches and exercises with the aim of preventing immobility. Physical therapy offers the following benefits to people who have muscle atrophy:

- preventing immobility;
- increasing muscle strength;
- improving circulation;
- reducing **spasticity**, which causes continuous muscle contraction.

Functional electric stimulation

Functional electrical stimulation (FES) is another effective treatment for muscle atrophy. It involves the use of electrical impulses to stimulate muscle contraction in affected muscles. During FES, a trained technician attaches electrodes to an atrophied limb. The electrodes transmit an electrical current, which triggers movement in the limb.

Focused ultrasound therapy

This technique delivers beams of ultrasound energy to specific areas in the body. The beams stimulate contractions in atrophied muscle tissue. This novel technology is in the development phase and has not yet entered the clinical trial phase.

Surgery

Surgical procedures may improve muscle function in people whose muscle atrophy is related to neurological conditions, injuries, or malnutrition.

Summary

Muscle atrophy, or muscle wasting, is characterized by a significant shortening of the muscle fibers and a loss of overall muscle mass. Several factors can contribute to muscle atrophy, such as:

- remaining immobile for long periods due to illness or injury;
- age;
- malnutrition;
- genetics;
- neurological problems;
- certain medical conditions, such as arthritis, myositis, ALS, and MS.

Treatment options will depend on each individual case, but they may include physical therapy, nutritional intervention, or surgery.

(1032 words)

muscle atrophy 肌肉萎缩

atrophied ['ætrəfɪd] *adj.* 萎缩的，衰退的
  v. 萎缩（atrophy 的过去分词）

lean [liːn] *adj.* 瘦且健康的，脂肪少的 *v.*
  倾斜，倚靠 *n.* 瘦肉；倾斜，倾斜度

irritable bowel syndrome 肠道易激综合征

celiac ['siːlɪˌæk] *adj.* 腹的，[解剖] 腹腔的

cachexia [kəˈkeksɪə] *n.* [内科] 恶病质；精
  神委顿

multiple sclerosis [内科] 多发性硬化

sarcopenia [sɑːkəʊˈpiːnɪə] *n.* 肌肉减少症，
  骨骼肌减少

frailty ['freɪlti] *n.* 虚弱，脆弱；意志薄弱

spinal muscular atrophy 脊髓性肌萎缩，脊
  肌萎缩症

chromosome ['krəʊməsəʊm] *n.* [遗] [细
  胞] 染色体

mutation [mjuːˈteɪʃn] *n.* 突变，变化

dystrophy ['dɪstrəfi] *n.* 营养障碍，营养失
  调，营养不良

amyotrophic [ˌæmɪəʊˈtrɒfɪk] *adj.* 肌萎缩
  的

lateral ['lætərəl] *adj.* 侧面的，横向的 *n.*
  侧部

amyotrophic lateral sclerosis 肌萎缩性侧
  束硬化症，肌萎缩侧索硬化

myositis [ˌmaɪəˈsaɪtɪs] *n.* [外科] 肌炎，肌
  肉发炎

polio ['pəʊlɪəʊ] *n.* 小 儿 麻 痹 症 （ =
  poliomyelitis），脊髓灰质炎

neurogenic [ˌnjʊərəʊˈdʒenɪk] *adj.* 神经源
  性的，起源于神经组织的

spasticity [spæsˈtɪsɪti] *n.* [临床] 痉挛状
  态，强直状态

◆ **Exercises**

Ⅰ. **Decide whether the following sentences are *True* or *False* according to the text.**

1. Long periods of inactivity and certain medical conditions are likely to develop muscle atrophy.

2. People with cachexia may experience a significant loss of appetite or weight loss, resulting in muscle atrophy.

3. Arthritis and myositis can contribute to muscle atrophy, but polio is unlikely to develop muscle atrophy.

4. Causes of muscle atrophy include poor nutrition, age, genetics, medical conditions as well as neurological problems.

5. Being inactive for a long period, difficulty balancing, limb weakness and limb smaller than the others are typical symptoms of muscle atrophy, but reduced muscle mass is not the symptom.

6. Functional electrical stimulation (FES) is the use of electrical impulses to stimulate muscle contraction in affected muscles. It is an effective treatment for muscle atrophy.

7. Physical therapy can prevent immobility, increase muscle strength, and improve circulation. However it can not reducing spasticity.

8. According to the text, focused ultrasound therapy has entered the clinical widespread use phase now.

9. Neurogenic muscle atrophy is caused by the damage to the nerves which control the muscles.

10. Spinal muscular atrophy (SMA) is a viral disorder that causes a loss of motor nerve cells and muscle atrophy.

Ⅱ. **Fill in the blanks with the proper form of words in the box.**

| sclerosis | mutation | myositis | atrophy | polio |
| cachexia | neurogenic | lean | sarcopenia | celiac |

1. _____ is a rare disease in which the muscle fibers and skin are inflamed and damaged, resulting in muscle weakness.

2. Many experts believe that vitiligo is the result of one or a combination of genetic, immunologic, biochemical and _____ factors.

3. _____ is a serious infectious disease that often makes people unable to use their legs.

4. If a copy of a gene is a bit different from the original, that's called a genetic _____.

5. The decline of growth hormone in the development of _____ is one of many factors, and its etiologic role needs to be demonstrated.

6. Multiple _____ is a potentially disabling disease of the brain and spinal cord (central nervous system).

7. _____ is general physical wasting and malnutrition usually associated with chronic disease.

8. If a muscle or other part of the body _____, it decreases in size or strength, often as a result of an illness.

9. It is a beautiful meat, very _____ and tender.

10. Men with untreated _____ disease may also have lower testosterone levels.

Ⅲ. **Translation: translate the passage into Chinese.**

Seven Brain Atrophy Causes That'll Go to Your Head

Brain atrophy is a wasting away of brain cells, or more accurately, the loss of brain neurons and the connections between them that are essential for functioning properly. This can result in communication difficulties, loss of muscle strength, seizures, and even more advanced problems such as dementia. Here are seven underlying causes of brain atrophy.

1. Traumatic Brain Injury

Livestrong.com notes that significant injuries to the head (and brain) can lead to brain atrophy. A traumatic brain injury can cause complications similar to a stroke by blocking blood flow to key areas of your brain, while also potentially causing direct brain tissue damage.

2. Huntington's Disease

This disorder is inherited and kills off brain cells, progressing from somewhat mild behavioral issues into full-blown problems such as difficulty walking and the inability to speak. Neuropathology-Web.org explains that the fatal condition usually shows up in middle age, but some people can get it before the age of 20. The source notes that certain areas of the brain of Huntington's patients are affected by atrophy.

3. Vitamin Deficiencies

You already know you need to eat a well-balanced diet with essential vitamins and nutrients to function at your best, but failing to do so may have more dire consequences, according to Medscape.com. It says a 2011 study found that a lack of Vitamin B_{12} in particular has been tied to brain atrophy.

4. Strokes

In the case of strokes, normal blood flow to your brain is interrupted. "The areas of the brain that do not receive blood begin to rapidly die, thus causing atrophy, potential cognitive deficits or death," explains Livestrong. com.

5. Heavy Drinking

The American Academy of Neurology announced in 2007 that alcohol abuse "shrinks" your brain. The findings came from a study of close to 2,000-brain scans of subjects aged 34 to 88, who ranged from non-drinkers, to moderate drinkers, to heavy drinkers.

6. Alzheimer's Disease

While this progressive disease is associated with wasting away of brain mass, affecting memory and even leading to death (usually from a related complication such as pneumonia), a post from ScienceDaily.com in 2009 notes that signs of brain atrophy on scans can predict progression to the deadly disease.

7. Aging

We were all aging, so there's not much we can do there. Livestrong.com explains that brain shrinkage is a part of normal aging, and that brains shrink at an average of 1.9 percent every 10 years.

(422 words)

IV. Give a presentation.

Dictate the causes, symptoms, treatments, etc. of Muscle Atrophy in English with 3—4 students. Try to use the formal expression, especially related medical terminology when you make your presentation.

V. Write an inquiry letter.

根据下列内容，写信咨询论文审稿情况。

论文《COVID-19 变异研究》已投稿超过 12 周了，并未收到任何回复，想咨询贵刊是否已有决定。

Text C

Rhabdomyolysis

Rhabdomyolysis is a serious syndrome due to a direct or indirect muscle injury. It results from the death of muscle fibers and release of their contents into the bloodstream. This can lead to serious complications such as renal (kidney) failure. This means the kidneys can not remove waste and concentrated urine. In rare cases, rhabdomyolysis can even cause death. However, prompt treatment often brings a good outcome. Here's what you need to know about rhabdomyolysis.

Causes

There are many traumatic and nontraumatic causes of rhabdomyolysis.

Traumatic causes of rhabdomyolysis include:

• A crush injury such as from an auto accident, fall, or building collapse;

• Long-lasting muscle compression such as that caused by prolonged immobilization after a fall or lying unconscious on a hard surface during illness or while under the influence of alcohol or medication;

• Electrical shock injury, lightning strike, or third-degree burn;

• **Venom** from a snake or insect bite.

Nontraumatic causes of rhabdomyolysis include:

• The use of alcohol or illegal drugs such as heroin, cocaine or amphetamines;

• Extreme muscle strain, especially in someone who is an untrained athlete; this can happen in elite athletes, too, and it can be more dangerous if there is more muscle mass to break down;

• The use of medications such as **antipsychotics** or statins, especially when given in high doses;

• A very high body temperature (**hyperthermia**) or heat stroke;

• Seizures or **delirium tremens**;

• A metabolic disorder such as **diabetic ketoacidosis**;

• Diseases of the muscles (**myopathy**) such as congenital muscle enzyme deficiency or Duchenne's muscular dystrophy;

• Viral infections such as the flu, HIV, or herpes simplex virus;

- Bacterial infections leading to toxins in tissues or the bloodstream (**sepsis**).

A previous history of rhabdomyolysis also increases the risk of having rhabdomyolysis again.

Signs and symptoms

Signs and symptoms of rhabdomyolysis may be hard to pinpoint. This is largely true because the course of rhabdomyolysis varies, depending on its cause. And, symptoms may occur in one area of the body or affect the whole body. Also, complications may occur in early and later stages.

The "classic **triad**" of rhabdomyolysis symptoms are: muscle pain in the shoulders, thighs, or lower back; muscle weakness or trouble moving arms and legs; and dark red or brown urine or decreased urination. Keep in mind that half of people with the condition may have no muscle-related symptoms.

Other common signs of rhabdomyolysis include:

- Abdominal pain;
- Nausea or vomiting;
- Fever, rapid heart rate;
- Confusion, dehydration, fever, or lack of consciousness.

Blood tests for **creatine kinase**, a product of muscle breakdown, and urine tests for **myoglobin**, a relative of hemoglobin that is released from damaged muscles, can help diagnose rhabdomyolysis (although in half of people with the condition, the myoglobin test may come up negative). Other tests may rule out other problems, confirm the cause of rhabdomyolysis, or check for complications.

Common complications of rhabdomyolysis include very high levels of potassium in the blood, which can lead to an irregular heartbeat or cardiac arrest and kidney damage (which occurs in up to half of patients). About one in four also develop problems with their liver. A condition called compartment syndrome may also occur after fluid resuscitation. This serious compression of nerves, blood vessels, and muscles can cause tissue damage and problems with blood flow.

Diagnosis

Rhabdomyolysis is suggested by the history of recent and past events and the physical examination. It is confirmed by blood and urine testing. An important part of diagnosing rhabdomyolysis is a comprehensive medical history and physical examination.

- The medical history may include questions about any medication use, drug and alcohol use, other medical conditions, any trauma or accident, etc. Blood tests include a complete blood count (CBC), a metabolic panel, muscle enzymes, and urinalysis.
- The levels of myoglobin can be elevated in blood and urine.
- The diagnosis of rhabdomyolysis is confirmed by detecting elevated muscle enzymes in blood, which include creatine phosphokinase (**CPK**), serum glutamic-oxaloacetic transaminase（**SGOT**）, serum glutamic phyuvic transaminase（**SGPT**）and Lactic Dehydrogenase（**LDH**）.
- The levels of these enzymes rise as the muscle is destroyed in rhabdomyolysis.

While the SGOT, SGPT, and LDH enzymes are found in muscles, they are more frequently associated with the liver. Therefore, elevations of SGOT and SGPT, without elevated CPK, are more typically indications of liver damage.

Of note, CPK is also in heart muscle (cardiac muscle) and brain. The laboratory is usually able to distinguish between the different components of this enzyme. For example, the fraction coming from skeletal muscle is referred to as CK-MM and the one from heart muscle is designated as CK-MB. There are small amounts of the CK-MB component in the skeletal muscle as well.

Treatment

Early diagnosis and treatment of rhabdomyolysis and its causes are keys to a successful outcome. You can expect full recovery with prompt treatment. Doctors can even reverse kidney damage. However, if compartment syndrome is not treated early enough, it may cause lasting damage.

If you have rhabdomyolysis, you will be admitted to the hospital to receive treatment for the cause. Treatment with intravenous (IV) fluids helps maintain urine production and prevent kidney failure. Rarely, dialysis treatment may be needed to help your kidneys filter waste products while they are recovering. Management of electrolyte abnormalities (potassium, calcium and **phosphorus**) helps protect your heart and other organs. You may also need a surgical procedure (**fasciotomy**) to relieve tension or pressure and loss of circulation if compartment syndrome threatens muscle death or nerve damage. In some cases, you may need to be in the intensive care unit (ICU) to allow close monitoring.

Most causes of rhabdomyolysis are reversible.

If rhabdomyolysis is related to a medical condition, such as diabetes or a thyroid disorder, appropriate treatment for the medical condition will be needed. And if rhabdomyolysis is related to a medication or drug, its use will need to be stopped or replaced with an alternative.

After treatment, discuss with your doctor any needed limitations on diet or activity. And, of course, avoid any potential causes of rhabdomyolysis in the future.

Complications

• One of the dreaded complications of rhabdomyolysis is kidney failure. This can occur for a variety of reasons. Direct injury to the kidney and plugging of the filtering tubes of the kidneys by the muscle proteins are among the causes of kidney function impairment in the setting of rhabdomyolysis.

• Another serious complication of rhabdomyolysis is called the compartment syndrome where muscle injury leads to swelling and increased pressure in a confined space (a compartment). This leads to compromised circulation which can endanger the affected tissue. The compartment syndrome is most common after injury in the lower legs, arms, or the muscles of the abdominal wall and can require emergency surgery.

• Rhabdomyolysis can also cause abnormality of electrolytes in the blood. Because of muscle injury, the contents of the muscle cells can be released into the blood causing high levels of potassium (**hyperkalemia**) and phosphorus (hyperphosphatemia).

(1173 words)

◇ **Vocabulary**

venom ['venəm] n. 毒液；恶意　vt. 使有毒，放毒

antipsychotic [ˌæntɪpsaɪˈʃɒtɪk] n. 抗精神病药

hyperthermia [ˌhaɪpəˈθɜːmɪə] n. 过高热，体温过高(= hyperpyrexia, hyperthermy)

delirium [dɪˈlɪrɪəm] n. 精神错乱，神志失常，说谵语状态

tremens [triːmenz] *n.* [医] 震颤，震动，震颤性谵妄

diabetic ketoacidosis [内科] 糖尿病酮症酸中毒，糖尿病酮酸症

myopathy [maɪˈɒpəθi] *n.* [外科] 肌病(复数 myopathies)

sepsis [ˈsepsɪs] *n.* [医] 败血症，脓毒病(复数 sepses)

triad [ˈtraɪæd] *n.* 三个一组，三人组合；三和音

creatine [ˈkriːətɪn] *n.* 肌(氨)酸

kinase [ˈkaɪneɪz] *n.* [生化] 激酶，致活酶

myoglobin [ˌmaɪəʊˈɡləʊbin] *n.* [生化] 肌红蛋白

CPK 肌酸磷酸激酶

SGOT 血清谷草转氨酶

SGPT 血清谷丙转氨酶

LDH 乳酸脱氢酶

phosphorus [ˈfɒsfərəs] *n.* 磷 (复数 phosphori 或 phosphoruses)

fasciotomy [fæʃɪˈɒtəmi] *n.* [外科] 筋膜切开术

hyperkalemia [haɪpəkeɪˈliːmiə] *n.* 高钾血，血钾过高

Text D

Congenital Myopathies

Congenital myopathies are rare muscle diseases mostly present at birth (congenital) that result from genetic defects. There are many different types of congenital myopathies, but most share common features, including lack of **muscle tone** and weakness.

Other signs and symptoms of some congenital myopathies include feeding and breathing difficulties, as well as skeletal conditions, such as **curvature** of the spine (**scoliosis**), weak bones (**osteopenia**) or hip problems. Signs and symptoms of congenital myopathies may not be apparent until later in infancy or childhood.

There are no known cures for congenital myopathies. However, the recent advances in gene therapy can provide treatment for congenital myopathies. The supportive treatments, including physical, occupational and speech therapies, nutritional support, and assisted breathing, may be helpful. Genetic counseling may help assess the risk of congenital myopathies in future pregnancies.

Symptoms

Signs and symptoms vary depending on the type of congenital myopathy. The severity of signs and symptoms also varies, though the conditions are often stable or slowly progressing.

Common signs and symptoms include:

- Lack of muscle tone;
- Muscle weakness;
- Delayed motor skills;
- Noticeable facial weakness;
- Drooping eyelids;
- **Muscle cramps** or contractions.

There are different types of congenital myopathies, some of which include:

- **Central core disease**. This condition causes muscle weakness and developmental problems. Some people may develop a significant reaction to general anesthesia (malignant hyperthermia).

• Centronuclear myopathies. These rare conditions cause muscle weakness in the face, arms, legs and eye muscles, and breathing problems.

• Congenital fiber type disproportion myopathy. Small fibers are found on muscle tissue during a biopsy. This condition causes muscle weakness in the face, neck, arms, legs and trunk.

• **Nemaline** myopathy. Nemaline myopathy is one of the more common congenital myopathies and causes muscle weakness in the face, neck, arms and legs, and sometimes scoliosis. It may also cause breathing and feeding problems.

• Multiminicore disease. This condition has several subtypes and often causes severe muscle weakness in the arms and legs, and scoliosis.

• **Myotubular** myopathy. This rare condition, which occurs only in males, causes muscle weakness, floppiness and breathing problems.

• Other myopathies. Other rare myopathies include **autophagic vacuolar** myopathy, cap disease, congenital myopathy with arrest of **myogenesis**, **myosin** storage (hyaline body) myopathy and zebra body myopathy.

Causes

Congenital myopathiesare caused by one or more genetic abnormalities in genes that control muscle development.

Risk factors

The only known risk factor for congenital myopathies is having a blood relative with one of these conditions, or one or both parents who carry a mutatedgene that causes them.

Complications

Congenital myopathies are associated with a number of complications, such as:

• Delays in motor skills;
• Scoliosis;
• Pneumonia;
• Respiratory failure;
• Feeding problems.

Prevention

There's no way to prevent congenital myopathies. If you're at high risk of having a child with a congenital myopathy, you may want to consult a genetic counselor before becoming pregnant.

A genetic counselor can help you understand your chances of having a child with a congenital myopathy. He or she can also explain the prenatal tests that are available and help explain the pros and cons of testing.

Diagnosis

To diagnose the condition, your doctor will review your medical and family history. He or she will conduct a physical and a neurological examination to find the cause of the muscle weakness and rule out other conditions. Your doctor may conduct several tests to diagnose congenital myopathy.

• Blood tests. These may be ordered to detect an enzyme called creatine kinase.

• Electromyography (EMG). Electromyography measures electrical activity within muscles.

• Genetic testing. This may be recommended to verify a particular mutation in a given gene.

• Muscle biopsy. A specialist may remove and examine a small sample of tissue (biopsy) from your muscle.

Prenatal diagnosis

If you have a known family history of congenital myopathies, you can opt for minimally invasive prenatal testing. **Chorionic villus** sampling can be done after 11 weeks of pregnancy. Amniocentesis can be done after 15 weeks, and **cordocentesis** can be done shortly after that. The risk of pregnancy loss associated with these tests is less than 1%.

Treatment

Congenital myopathies can't be cured, but doctors can help you manage the condition and symptoms. Treatment may include several options.

• Genetic counseling. Genetic counselors may help you understand the genetics of the condition.

• Medications. Medications may help treat symptoms of some myopathies. For example, the drug **albuterol** (Proair HFA, Ventolin HFA, others) may be helpful in some congenital myopathies.

• Nutritional and respiratory support. Nutritional or respiratory support may be needed as the condition progresses.

• Orthopedic treatments. Orthopedic support devices or other treatments, such as surgery to correct or improve scoliosis or contractures, may be helpful.

• Physical, occupational or speech therapy. Physical, occupational or speech therapy may help manage symptoms. Low-impact aerobic exercise, such as walking and swimming, can help maintain strength, mobility and general health. Some types of strengthening exercises also might be helpful.

• Respiratory therapy. Some patients need respiratory support or respiratory treatments.

In addition to these treatments, some people with congenital myopathies may benefit from an evaluation from an endocrinologist. An endocrinologist can monitor bone health, as bone diseases such as osteopenia and osteoporosis may develop in some people with congenital myopathies.

It's also important to take precautions to prevent respiratory infections. Annual influenza vaccinations and regular pneumonia vaccinations are recommended. Try to avoid contact with anyone who has an obvious respiratory infection.

(910 words)

◆ Vocabulary

congenital myopathy 先天性肌病
muscle tone 肌张力，肌肉紧张度
curvature [ˈkɜːvətʃə(r)] n. 弯曲，[数] 曲率
scoliosis [ˌskəʊliˈəʊsɪs] n. [外科] 脊柱侧凸
osteopenia [ˌɒstɪəʊˈpiːnɪə] n. 骨量减少，骨质缺乏
muscle cramps 肌肉痉挛
central core disease 中央轴突症，中央轴空病
nemaline [niːməˈlɪn] n. 纤维质，纤维状
myotubular [maɪətˈjuːbjʊlə] adj. 肌管的

autophagic [ɔːtəˈfægɪk] adj. 自体吞噬的
vacuolar [vækjuˈəʊlər] adj. 空泡的，有液泡的
myogenesis [maˈɪuːdʒenəsɪs] n. 肌生成，肌细胞生成
myosin [ˈmaɪə(ʊ)sɪn] n. [生化]肌浆球蛋白，肌球蛋白，肌凝蛋白
chorionic [kəʊriˈɒnɪk] adj. 绒(毛)膜的
villus [ˈvɪləs] n. 绒毛；长茸毛
cordocentesis [kɔːdəʊsentɪzɪs] 脐穿刺
albuterol [ælbˈjʊtərəl] n. 沙丁胺醇，舒喘宁

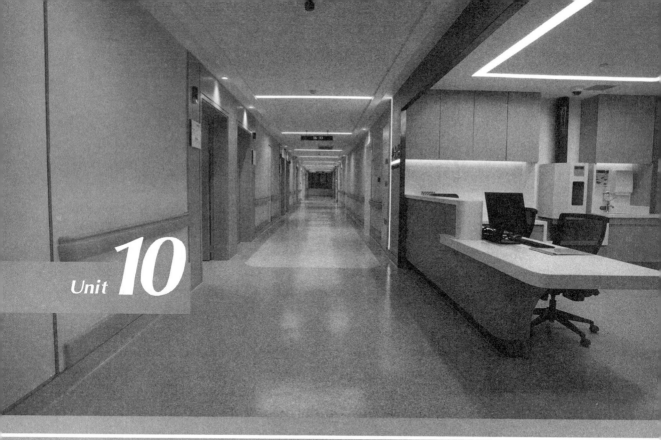

Some Common Diseases of the Immune System

✓参考答案
✓微课等资源

Text A

Rheumatoid Arthritis

Rheumatoid arthritis is a chronic inflammatory disorder that can affect more than just your joints. In some people, the condition can damage a wide variety of body systems, including the skin, eyes, lungs, heart and blood vessels. An autoimmune disorder, rheumatoid arthritis occurs when your immune system mistakenly attacks your own body's tissues. Unlike the wear-and-tear damage of osteoarthritis, rheumatoid arthritis affects the lining of your joints, causing a painful swelling that can eventually result in bone erosion and joint deformity. The inflammation associated with rheumatoid arthritis is what can damage other parts of the body as well. While new types of medications have improved treatment options dramatically, severe rheumatoid arthritis can still cause physical disabilities.

Symptoms

Signs and symptoms of rheumatoid arthritis may include:

• Tender, warm, swollen joints;
• Joint stiffness that is usually worse in the mornings and after inactivity;
• Fatigue, fever and loss of appetite.

Early rheumatoid arthritis tends to affect your smaller joints first—particularly the joints that attach your fingers to your hands and your toes to your feet. As the disease progresses, symptoms often spread to the wrists, knees, ankles, elbows, hips and shoulders. In most cases, symptoms occur in the same joints on both sides of your body.

About 40% of people who have rheumatoid arthritis also experience signs and symptoms that don't involve the joints. Areas that may be affected include:

• Skin;
• Eyes;
• Lungs;
• Heart;
• Kidneys;

- Salivary glands;
- Nerve tissue;
- Bone marrow;
- Blood vessels.

Rheumatoid arthritis signs and symptoms may vary in severity and may even come and go. Periods of increased disease activity, called flares, alternate with periods of relative remission—when the swelling and pain fade or disappear. Over time, rheumatoid arthritis can cause joints to deform and shift out of place.

Causes

Rheumatoid arthritis is an autoimmune disease. Normally, your immune system helps protect your body from infection and disease. In rheumatoid arthritis, your immune system attacks healthy tissue in your joints. It can also cause medical problems with your heart, lungs, nerves, eyes and skin.

Doctors don't know what starts this process, although a genetic component appears likely. While your genes don't actually cause rheumatoid arthritis, they can make you more likely to react to environmental factors— such as infection with certain viruses and bacteria—that may trigger the disease.

Diagnosis

Rheumatoid arthritis can be difficult to diagnose in its early stages because the early signs and symptoms mimic those of many other diseases. There is no one blood test or physical finding to confirm the diagnosis. During the physical exam, your doctor will check your joints for swelling, redness and warmth. He or she may also check your reflexes and muscle strength.

Blood tests

People with rheumatoid arthritis often have an elevated erythrocyte sedimentation rate (ESR, also known as sed rate) or C-reactive protein (CRP) level, which may indicate the presence of an inflammatory process in the body. Other common blood tests look for rheumatoid factor and anticyclic citrullinated **peptide** (anti-CCP) antibodies.

Imaging tests

Your doctor may recommend X-rays to help track the progression of rheumatoid arthritis in your joints over time. MRI and ultrasound tests can help your doctor judge the severity of the disease in your body.

Treatment

There is no cure for rheumatoid arthritis. But clinical studies indicate that remission of symptoms is more likely when treatment begins early with medications known as disease-modifying antirheumatic drugs (DMARDs).

Medications

The types of medications recommended by your doctor will depend on the severity of your symptoms and how long you've had rheumatoid arthritis.

- NSAIDs. Nonsteroidal anti-inflammatory drugs (NSAIDs) can relieve pain and reduce inflammation. Over-the-counter NSAIDs include ibuprofen (Advil, Motrin IB, others) and naproxen sodium (Aleve). Stronger NSAIDs are available by prescription. Side effects may include stomach irritation, heart problems and kidney damage.

- Steroids. Corticosteroid medications, such as prednisone, reduce inflammation and pain and slow joint damage. Side effects may include thinning of bones, weight gain and diabetes. Doctors often prescribe a corticosteroid to relieve symptoms quickly, with the goal of gradually tapering off the medication.

- Conventional DMARDs. These drugs can slow the progression of rheumatoid arthritis and save the joints and other tissues from permanent damage. Common DMARDs include **methotrexate** (Trexall, Otrexup, others), **leflunomide** (Arava), **hydroxychloroquine** (Plaquenil) and **sulfasalazine** (Azulfidine). Side effects vary but may include liver damage and severe lung infections.

- Biologic agents. Also known as biologic response modifiers, this newer class of DMARDs includes abatacept, **adalimumab**, **anakinra**, certolizumab, **etanercept**, **golimumab**, **infliximab**, **rituximab**, sarilumab and tocilizumab. Biologic DMARDs are usually most effective when paired with a conventional DMARD, such as methotrexate. This type of drug also increases the risk of infections.

- Targeted synthetic DMARDs. Baricitinib, tofacitinib and upadacitinib may be used if conventional DMARDs and biologics haven't been effective. Higher doses of tofacitinib can increase the risk of blood clots in the lungs, serious heart-related events and cancer.

Therapy

Your doctor may refer you to a physical or occupational therapist who can teach you exercises to help keep your joints flexible. The therapist may also suggest new ways to do daily tasks that will be easier on your joints. For example, you may want to pick up an object using your forearms.

Assistive devices can make it easier to avoid stressing your painful joints. For instance, a kitchen knife equipped with a hand grip helps protect your finger and wrist joints. Certain tools, such as buttonhooks, can make it easier to get dressed. Catalogs and medical supply stores are good places to look for ideas.

Surgery

If medications fail to prevent or slow joint damage, you and your doctor may consider surgery to repair damaged joints. Surgery may help restore your ability to use your joint. It can also reduce pain and improve function. Rheumatoid arthritis surgery may involve one or more of the following procedures:

• **Synovectomy**. Surgery to remove the inflamed lining of the joint (synovium) can help reduce pain and improve the joint's flexibility.

• Tendon repair. Inflammation and joint damage may cause tendons around your joint to loosen or rupture. Your surgeon may be able to repair the tendons around your joint.

• Joint fusion. Surgically fusing a joint may be recommended to stabilize or realign a joint and for pain relief when a joint replacement isn't an option.

• Total joint replacement. During joint replacement surgery, your surgeon removes the damaged parts of your joint and inserts a **prosthesis** made of metal and plastic.

Surgery carries a risk of bleeding, infection and pain. Discuss the benefits and risks with your doctor.

Lifestyle and home remedies

You can take steps to care for your body if you have rheumatoid arthritis. These self-care measures, when used along with your rheumatoid arthritis medications, can help you manage your signs and symptoms:

• Exercise regularly. Gentle exercise can help strengthen the muscles around your joints, and it can help reduce fatigue you might feel. Check with your doctor before you start exercising. If you're just getting started, begin by taking a walk. Avoid exercising tender, injured or severely inflamed joints.

• Apply heat or cold. Heat can help ease your pain and relax tense, painful muscles. Cold may dull the sensation of pain. Cold also has a numbing effect and can reduce swelling.

　　• Relax. Find ways to cope with pain by reducing stress in your life. Techniques such as guided imagery, deep breathing and muscle relaxation can all be used to control pain.

(1251 words)

Vocabulary

rheumatoid arthritis 类风湿性关节炎

peptide ['peptaɪd] n. 肽

methotrexate [ˌmeθəʊ'trekseɪt] n. 甲氨蝶呤，[药] 氨甲叶酸，氨甲蝶呤

leflunomide ['leflʌnɒmaɪd] n. 来氟米特

hydroxychloroquine [haɪ'drɑːksɪ'klɔːrəkwiːn] n. [药] 羟化氯喹

sulfasalazine [sʌlfə'sæləzɪn] n. 柳氮磺胺吡啶

adalimumab [ædælɪmjuː'mæb] [医] 阿达木单抗 (免疫调节药)

anakinra [ɑː'neɪkɪnrə] n. [医] 阿那白滞素 (白介素受体阻滞药)

etanercept [eɪtənə'sept] n. [药] 依那西普

golimumab n. [药] 戈利木单抗

infliximab [ɪnf'lɪksɪmæb] n. [医] 英夫利昔单抗 (抗类风湿药)

rituximab [rɪtəksɪ'mæb] n. [医] 利妥昔单抗 (抗肿瘤药)

synovectomy [sɪnə'vektəmi] n. 滑膜切除术

prosthesis [prɒs'θiːsɪs] n. 假体；假肢

Exercises

Ⅰ. Decide whether the following sentences are *True* or *False* according to the text.

1. Rheumatoid arthritis is an acute inflammatory disorder that can affect more than your joints.

2. As an autoimmune disorder, rheumatoid arthritis occurs when your immune system mistakenly attacks your own body's tissues.

3. Rheumatoid arthritis only affects the lining of your joints, without causing bone erosion.

4. Early rheumatoid arthritis tends to affect the smaller joints first, then often spread to the wrists, ankles, etc.

5. Rheumatoid arthritis can cause joints to deform and shift out of place eventually.

6. Doctors already know the cause of rheumatoid arthritis, that is the genetic component.

7. People with rheumatoid arthritis often have a lower erythrocyte sedimentation rate

or C-reactive protein level.

8. MRI, not ultrasound tests can help your doctor judge the severity of your rheumatoid arthritis.

9. Different degrees of rheumatoid arthritis will take different types of medications.

10. If medications don't work well, surgery may be recommended by your doctor to treat rheumatoid arthritis.

II. **Fill in the blanks with the proper form of words in the box.**

synovectomy	corticosteroid	therapist	joint	rheumatoid
prosthesis	tendon	salivary	arthritis	sedimentation

1. _____ refers to inflammation of a joint or joints.

2. _____ arthritis is a painful condition that affects your joints.

3. _____ with arthroscopy can remove the pathological synovial membrane.

4. There is some _____ in the ink.

5. While playing badminton, I ruptured my Achilles _____.

6. _____ is a steroid hormone produced by the adrenal cortex or synthesized.

7. A _____ is an artificial body part that is used to replace a natural part.

8. A _____ is a person who is skilled in a particular type of therapy, especially psychotherapy.

9. A _____ refers to the point of connection between two bones or elements of a skeleton.

10. The saliva in our mouths is secreted from the _____ gland.

III. **Translation: translate the passage into Chinese.**

Gout is a common and complex form of arthritis that can affect anyone. It's characterized by sudden, severe attacks of pain, swelling, redness and tenderness in one or more joints, most often in the big toe. An attack of gout can occur suddenly, often waking you up in the middle of the night with the sensation that your big toe is on fire. The affected joint is hot, swollen and so tender that even the weight of the bedsheet on it may seem intolerable. Gout symptoms may come and go, but there are ways to manage symptoms and prevent flares.

Symptoms

The signs and symptoms of gout almost always occur suddenly, and often at night. They include:

• Intense joint pain. Gout usually affects the big toe, but it can occur in any joint. Other commonly affected joints include the ankles, knees, elbows, wrists and fingers. The pain is likely to be most severe within the first 4 to 12 hours after it begins.

- Lingering discomfort. After the most severe pain subsides, some joint discomfort may last from a few days to a few weeks. Later attacks are likely to last longer and affect more joints.

- Inflammation and redness. The affected joint or joints become swollen, tender, warm and red.

- Limited range of motion. As gout progresses, you may not be able to move your joints normally.

Causes

Gout occurs when urate crystals accumulate in your joint, causing the inflammation and intense pain of a gout attack. Urate crystals can form when you have high levels of uric acid in your blood. Your body produces uric acid when it breaks down purines—substances that are found naturally in your body.

Purines are also found in certain foods, including red meat and organ meats, such as liver. Purine-rich seafood includes anchovies, sardines, mussels, scallops, trout and tuna. Alcoholic beverages, especially beer, and drinks sweetened with fruit sugar promote higher levels of uric acid.

Normally, uric acid dissolves in your blood and passes through your kidneys into your urine. But sometimes either your body produces too much uric acid or your kidneys excrete too little uric acid. When this happens, uric acid can build up, forming sharp, needle-like urate crystals in a joint or surrounding tissue that cause pain, inflammation and swelling.

(382 words)

Ⅳ. Give a presentation.

Dictate the causes, symptoms, treatments, etc. of Rheumatoid Arthritis in English with 3—4 students. Try to use the formal expression when you make your presentation.

Ⅴ. Write a letter of invitation.

根据下列内容,写一份报告邀请信。

怀特先生邀请希尔先生于 10 月 23 日(星期日)早上 8:30 在讲座厅作有关牙科学的报告,题目自拟。听众是我院所有的牙科医生和在我科室的实习生。

Text B

Sjogren's Syndrome

Sjogren's syndrome is an autoimmune disease that causes your immune system to go **haywire** and attack healthy cells instead of invading bacteria or viruses. Your white blood cells, which normally protect you from germs, attack the glands that are in charge of making moisture. When that happens, they can't produce tears and saliva, so your eyes, mouth, and other parts of your body dry out. There are treatments that bring relief, though.

It's natural to worry when you learn you've got a lifelong disease that will need regular care. Keep in mind that most people with Sjogren's stay healthy and don't have serious problems. You should be able to keep doing all the things you love to do without making many changes.

Causes and risk factors

Doctors don't know the exact cause. You may have genes that put you at risk. An infection with a bacteria or virus may be a trigger that sets the disease in motion. For example, let's say you have a defective gene that's linked to Sjogren's, and then you get an infection. Your immune system swings into action.

White blood cells normally lead the attack against the germs. But because of your faulty gene, your white blood cells target healthy cells in the glands that make saliva and tears. There's no let-up in the fight, so your symptoms will keep going unless you get treatment.

Some other things can make you more likely to have Sjogren's, including:

• Age. Sjogren's usually affects people over 40, but younger adults and children can get it, too.
• Gender. Women are 10 times more likely to have Sjogren's than men.
• Other autoimmune issues. Nearly half of all people who have Sjogren's also have another autoimmune condition, like lupus and rheumatoid arthritis.

Symptoms

The symptoms of Sjogren's can be different from person to person. You may have just one or two, or you may have many. By far, the most common symptoms are:

- Dry mouth that may have a chalky or cotlon feeling;
- Dry eyes that may burn, itch, or feel **gritty**;
- Dry throat, lips, or skin;
- Dryness in your nose;
- A change in taste or smell;
- Swollen glands in your neck and face;
- Skin rashes and sensitivity to **UV light**;
- Dry cough or shortness of breath;
- Feeling tired;
- Trouble concentrating or remembering things;
- Headache;
- Dryness in the vagina in women;
- Swelling, pain, and stiffness in your joints;
- Heartburn, a sensation of burning that moves from your stomach to your chest;
- Numbness or tingling in some parts of your body.

Diagnosis

Because so many people with Sjogren's also have another autoimmune disease, and Sjogren's symptoms sometimes look a lot like some other diseases, like **fibromyalgia** or chronic fatigue syndrome, it can sometimes be hard for your doctor to give you a diagnosis.

To get clues, your doctor will give you a physical exam and may ask you questions such as:

- Do your eyes itch or burn often?
- Are you getting a lot of cavities in your teeth?
- Does your mouth get dry? How about your lips?
- Do you have stiff or painful joints?

Your doctor may ask you to get some blood tests. They will take some blood from your vein and send it to a lab to get checked.

The blood tests measure the levels of the different types of blood cells you have and can show if you have germ-fighting proteins (antibodies) that many people with Sjogren's have. They can also measure inflammation in your body and the amount of certain proteins called **immunoglobulins** that are part of your body's infection-fighting system. High levels of these can be signs that you have the disease.

Your blood tests can also give your doctor an idea of how well your liver is working and show if there might be any issues with it.

Your doctor also may recommend a few tests related to your eyes and mouth:

• Schirmer tear test. This measures how dry your eyes are. Your doctor will put a small piece of paper under your lower eyelid to see how much your eye tears up.

• **Slit lamp**. Your doctor uses this magnifying device to get a close look at the surface of your eyes.

• Dye tests. Your doctor puts drops of dye in your eyes to check for dry spots.

• Salivary flow test. This measures the amount of saliva you make over a certain amount of time.

• Salivary gland biopsy. Your doctor will take a tiny piece of a salivary gland, usually from your lower lip, for testing. This can tell them if you have a rare condition called **lymphocytic infiltrate**, which is a buildup of white blood cells that look like bumps.

In some cases, they also may suggest an imaging test:

• **Sialogram**. Your doctor uses this to show how much saliva flows into your mouth. They'll give you a shot of dye in the salivary glands in front of your ears and use a special kind of X-ray to take pictures of its flow.

• Salivary **scintigraphy**. This imaging test is used to track how quickly a tiny amount of a radioactive substance gets to all of your salivary glands. Your doctor will give you a shot of the substance then track its progress over the next hour.

Treatment

You'll need to take medicine throughout your life to help you manage your symptoms. You can buy some kinds in a drugstore without a prescription, while your doctor may need to prescribe stronger ones if those don't work well enough.

For instance, drops called "artificial tears" can keep your eyes from drying out. You'll need to use them regularly throughout the day. There are also gels that you put on your eyes at night. The advantage of the gels is that they stick to your eye's surface, so you won't need to apply them as often as the drops.

If artificial tears aren't helping, your doctor may prescribe drugs for your dry eyes, including:

- Cequa;
- Lacrisert;
- Restasis.

Lacrisert is a tiny rod-shaped medicine. You put it into your eye with a special applicator, usually once or twice a day. Cequa and Restasis come in drops, which you use twice a day.

Another treatment option for dry eyes is a procedure called punctal **occlusion**. This is when your doctor puts tiny plugs into your tear ducts to block them up. This keeps tears from draining away too fast, meaning they stay on your eyes longer and help your eyes stay moist.

To help your dry mouth, your doctor may prescribe drugs that boost the amount of your saliva, including:

- Cevimeline;
- Supersaturated calcium phosphate rinse;
- Pilocarpine.

There are other treatments for some of the less common symptoms of Sjogren's syndrome. For instance, if you get yeast infections in your mouth, your doctor might prescribe antifungal medicine.

If you get heartburn, your doctor may give you medicines that **curb** the amount of acid in your stomach.

Your doctor may also suggest a medicine called hydroxychloroquine (Plaquenil) to treat your joint pain. It's a drug that's also used to treat malaria, lupus, and rheumatoid arthritis.

It's rare, but some people with Sjogren's get symptoms throughout the body, including belly pain, fever, rashes, or lung and kidney problems. For those situations, doctors sometimes prescribe prednisone (a steroid) or an anti-inflammation drug called methotrexate (Rheumatrex, Trexall).

(1268 words)

Vocabulary

Sjogren's syndrome 干燥综合征

haywire ['heɪˌwaɪə(r)] adj. 乱七八糟的，失去控制的，故障 n. 捆干草用的铁丝

gritty ['grɪti] adj. 有沙砾的；多沙的

UV light 紫外光；紫外线

fibromyalgia [ˌfaɪbrəʊmaɪ'ældʒiːə] n. 纤维性肌痛，纤维肌痛

immunoglobulin [ˌɪmjʊnəʊ'glɒbjʊlɪn] n. [生化]免疫球蛋白

slit lamp 缝灯，狭缝灯，裂隙灯

lymphocytic [ˌlɪmfə'saɪtɪk] adj. [解]淋巴球的；淋巴细胞的

infiltrate ['ɪnfɪltreɪt] v. (使)渗透，(使)渗入 n. (医学)浸润物

sialogram [sjəlɒg'ræm] n. 涎管 X 线造影片，涎管 X 线片

scintigraphy [ˌsɪn'tɪgrəfi] n. 闪烁扫描术；闪烁法

occlusion [ə'kluːʒn] n. 闭塞；吸收

curb [kɜːb] vt. 抑制；勒住 n. 路边；克制；勒马绳

Exercises

Ⅰ. **Decide whether the following sentences are *True* or *False* according to the text.**

1. Sjogren's syndrome is an autoimmune disease that your glands can't produce enough tears and saliva.

2. Most people with Sjogren's don't stay healthy and have serious problems.

3. Although the exact cause of Sjogren's syndrome isn't clear, genes may put you at risk.

4. Gender and age are the risk factors of Sjogren's syndrome.

5. The common symptoms of Sjogren's syndrome include dry eyes, mouth, throat and cough.

6. Many people with Sjogren's also have another autoimmune disease.

7. The blood tests can't measure inflammation in your body and the amount of immunoglobulins.

8. Slit lamp measures how dry your eyes are.

9. Headache, heartburn and numbness are the common symptoms of Sjogren's syndrome.

10. Men are 10 times more likely to have Sjogren's than women.

Ⅱ. **Fill in the blanks with the proper form of words in the box.**

cavity	immunoglobulin	syndrome	lupus	bump
antibody	fibromyalgia	vagina	gland	malaria

1. _____ lies in the lower part of the female reproductive tract.

2. Persons with _____ typically experience long-lasting or chronic pain, as well as muscle stiffness and tenderness.

3. I have a toothache because there is a(n) _____ in one of my teeth.

4. _____ is a class of proteins produced in lymph tissue in vertebrates and that function as antibodies in the immune response.

5. Infection can cause a(n) _____ flare.

6. _____ is a number of symptoms that belong to a specific disease.

7. _____ are substances that a person's or an animal's body produces in their blood in order to destroy substances that carry disease.

8. _____ is something that bulges out or is protuberant or projects from its surroundings.

9. The prostate is a small _____ in men.

10. _____ is a disease marked by recurring chills and fever and caused by a parasite carried by a mosquito.

III. Translation: translate the passage into Chinese.

Dermatomyositis is an uncommon inflammatory disease marked by muscle weakness and a distinctive skin rash. The condition can affect adults and children. In adults, dermatomyositis usually occurs in the late 40s to early 60s. In children, it most often appears between 5 and 15 years of age. Dermatomyositis affects more females than males. There's no cure for dermatomyositis, but periods of symptom improvement can occur. Treatment can help clear the skin rash and help you regain muscle strength and function.

Symptoms

The signs and symptoms of dermatomyositis can appear suddenly or develop gradually over time. The most common signs and symptoms include:

• Skin changes. A violet-colored or dusky red rash develops, most commonly on your face and eyelids and on your knuckles, elbows, knees, chest and back. The rash, which can be itchy and painful, is often the first sign of dermatomyositis.

• Muscle weakness. Progressive muscle weakness involves the muscles closest to the trunk, such as those in your hips, thighs, shoulders, upper arms and neck. The weakness affects both the left and right sides of your body, and tends to gradually worsen.

Causes

The cause of dermatomyositis is unknown, but the disease has much in common with autoimmune disorders, in which your immune system mistakenly attacks your body tissues.

Genetic and environmental factors also might play a role. Environmental factors could include viral infections, sun exposure, certain medications and smoking.

Complications

Possible complications of dermatomyositis include:

• Difficulty swallowing. If the muscles in your esophagus are affected, you can have problems swallowing, which can cause weight loss and malnutrition.

• Aspiration pneumonia. Difficulty swallowing can also cause you to breathe food or liquids, including saliva, into your lungs.

• Breathing problems. If the condition affects your chest muscles, you might have breathing problems, such as shortness of breath.

• Calcium deposits. These can occur in your muscles, skin and connective tissues as the disease progresses. These deposits are more common in children with dermatomyositis and develop earlier in the course of the disease.

(334 words)

IV. Give a presentation.

Dictate the causes, symptoms, treatments, etc. of Sjogren's Syndrome in English with 3—4 students. Try to use the formal expression, especially related medical terminology when you make your presentation.

V. Write a letter of acceptance.

根据下列内容写一封接受邀请的回信。

非常感谢李涛教授邀请我参加将于 4 月 20—23 日在北京举行的癌症国际论坛。我接受邀请并将在规定的日期前将会议论文发送到论文委员会，预祝大会取得成功。

Text C

Systemic Lupus Erythematosus

Systemic lupus erythematous (SLE), is the most common type of lupus. SLE is an autoimmune disease in which the immune system attacks its own tissues, causing widespread inflammation and tissue damage in the affected organs. It can affect the joints, skin, brain, lungs, kidneys, and blood vessels. There is no cure for lupus, but medical interventions and lifestyle changes can help control it.

Seriousness

The seriousness of SLE can range from mild to life-threatening. The disease should be treated by a doctor or a team of doctors who specialize in care of SLE patients. People with lupus that get proper medical care, preventive care, and education can significantly improve function and quality of life.

Causes

The causes of SLE are unknown, but are believed to be linked to environmental, genetic, and hormonal factors.

Signs and symptoms

People with SLE may experience a variety of symptoms that include fatigue, skin rashes, fevers, and pain or swelling in the joints. Among some adults, having a period of SLE symptoms—called flares—may happen every so often, sometimes even years apart, and go away at other times—called remission. However, other adults may experience SLE flares more frequently throughout their life. Other symptoms can include sun sensitivity, oral ulcers, arthritis, lung problems, heart problems, kidney problems, seizures, **psychosis**, and blood cell and immunological abnormalities.

Complications

SLE can have both short- and long-term effects on a person's life. Early diagnosis and effective treatments can help reduce the damaging effects of SLE and improve the chance to have better function and quality of life. Poor access to care, late diagnosis, less effective treatments, and poor adherence to therapeutic regimens may increase the damaging effects of SLE, causing more complications and an increased risk of death.

SLE can limit a person's physical, mental, and social functioning. These limitations experienced by people with SLE can impact their quality of life, especially if they experience fatigue. Fatigue is the most common symptom negatively affecting the quality of life of people with SLE.

Many studies use employment as a measure to determine the quality of life of people with SLE, as employment is central to a person's life. Some studies have shown that the longer a person has had SLE, the less likely they are to be a part of the workforce. On average, only 46% of people with SLE of working age report being employed.

Adherence to treatment **regimens** is often a problem, especially among young women of childbearing age (15 to 44 years). Because SLE treatment may require the use of strong immunosuppressive medications that can have serious side effects, female patients must stop taking the medication before and during pregnancy to protect unborn children from harm.

Diagnosis

SLE is diagnosed by a health care provider using symptom assessments, physical examination, X-rays, and lab tests. SLE may be difficult to diagnose because its early signs and symptoms are not specific and can look like signs and symptoms of other diseases. SLE may also be misdiagnosed if only a blood test is used for diagnosis. Because diagnosis can be challenging, it is important to see a doctor specializing in **rheumatology** for a final diagnosis. Rheumatologists sometimes use specific criteria to classify SLE for research purposes.

Risk factors

SLE can affect people of all ages, including children. However, women of childbearing ages—15 to 44 years—are at greatest risk of developing SLE. Women of all ages are affected far more than men (estimates range from 4 to 12 women for every 1 man).

Treatment

Treating SLE often requires a team approach because of the number of organs that can be affected.

SLE treatment consists primarily of immunosuppressive drugs that inhibit activity of the immune system. Hydroxychloroquine and corticosteroids (e. g., prednisone) are often used to treat SLE. The FDA approved **belimumab** in 2011, the first new drug for SLE in more than 50 years.

SLE also may occur with other autoimmune conditions that require additional treatments, like Sjogren's syndrome, antiphospholipid syndrome, thyroiditis, hemolytic anemia, and idiopathic thrombocytopenia purpura.

Incidence and prevalence

Incidence and prevalence are terms commonly used to describe how many people have a disease or condition.

CDC uses the latest available data for important research questions. Recent national estimates of prevalence and incidence are not available for SLE. SLE is relatively uncommon, is difficult to diagnose, and is not a reportable disease, so it is expensive to capture all diagnosed cases reliably for epidemiologic studies. There are no recent studies to determine if SLE prevalence or incidence are changing over time.

CDC funded several population-based patient registries to better estimate how many people have doctor-diagnosed SLE in certain racial/ ethnic groups. The registries provide the most recent available prevalence and incidence estimates for SLE for whites, blacks, and American Indians/ Alaska Natives was published in 2014. The CDC-funded lupus registries used similar intensive methods for case finding (hospitals, specialists' practices, health department data) and for seeing if possible cases met standard classification criteria (i.e., medical record review). See the Lupus Studies page for more information.

Death

Causes of premature death associated with SLE are mainly active disease, organ failure (e. g., kidneys), infection, or cardiovascular disease from accelerated atherosclerosis. In a large international SLE cohort with average follow-up of over 8 years during an observation interval, observed deaths were much higher than expected for all causes, and in particular for circulatory disease, infections, renal disease, and some cancers. Those who were female, younger, and had SLE of short duration were at higher risk of SLE-associated mortality.

Using death certificates for US residents, SLE was identified as the underlying cause of death for an average of 1,176 deaths per year from 2010 to 2016. SLE was identified as a contributing cause of death (one of multiple causes of death, including underlying cause of death) for an average of 2,061 deaths per year during that 7-year-period.

（1021 words）

◇ **Vocabulary**

systemic lupus erythematosus 系统性红斑
　狼疮
erythematosus [erɪˌθiːməˈtəʊsəs] *n.* 全身性
　红斑狼疮 *adj.* 红斑的

psychosis [saɪˈkəʊsɪs] *n.* 精神病，精神错乱
regimen [ˈredʒɪmən] *n.* [医] 养生法
rheumatology [ˌruːməˈtɒlədʒi] *n.* 风湿病学
belimumab 贝利单抗

Text D

Ankylosing Spondylitis

Ankylosing spondylitis is an inflammatory disease that, over time, can cause some of the bones in the spine to **fuse**. This fusing makes the spine less flexible and can result in a **hunched** posture. If ribs are affected, it can be difficult to breathe deeply.

Ankylosing spondylitis affects men more often than women. Signs and symptoms typically begin in early adulthood. Inflammation can also occur in other parts of the body—most commonly, the eyes.

There is no cure for ankylosing spondylitis, but treatments can lessen symptoms and possibly slow progression of the disease.

Symptoms

Early signs and symptoms of ankylosing spondylitis might include pain and stiffness in the lower back and hips, especially in the morning and after periods of inactivity. Neck pain and fatigue also are common. Over time, symptoms might worsen, improve or stop at irregular intervals.

The areas most commonly affected are:

- The joint between the base of the spine and the pelvis;
- The vertebrae in the lower back;
- The places where tendons and ligaments attach to bones, mainly in the spine, but sometimes along the back of the heel;
- The cartilage between the breastbone and the ribs;
- The hip and shoulder joints.

Causes

Ankylosing spondylitis has no known specific cause, though genetic factors seem to be involved. In particular, people who have a gene called HLA-B27 are at a greatly increased risk of developing ankylosing spondylitis. However, only some people with the gene develop the condition.

Risk factors

Men are more likely to develop ankylosing spondylitis than are women.

Onset generally occurs in late adolescence or early adulthood. Most people who have ankylosing spondylitis have the HLA-B27 gene. But many people who have this gene never develop ankylosing spondylitis.

Complications

In severe ankylosing spondylitis, new bone forms as part of the body's attempt to heal. This new bone gradually bridges the gap between vertebrae and eventually fuses sections of vertebrae. Those parts of the spine become stiff and inflexible. Fusion can also stiffen the rib cage, restricting lung capacity and function.

Other complications might include:

• Eye inflammation (**uveitis**). One of the most common complications of ankylosing spondylitis, uveitis can cause rapid-onset eye pain, sensitivity to light and blurred vision. See your doctor right away if you develop these symptoms.

• Compression fractures. Some people's bones weaken during the early stages of ankylosing spondylitis. Weakened vertebrae can **crumple**, increasing the severity of a stooped posture. Vertebral fractures can put pressure on and possibly injure the spinal cord and the nerves that pass through the spine.

• Heart problems. Ankylosing spondylitis can cause problems with the aorta, the largest artery in the body. The inflamed aorta can enlarge to the point that it distorts the shape of the aortic valve in the heart, which impairs its function. The inflammation associated with ankylosing spondylitis increases the risk of heart disease in general.

Diagnosis

During the physical exam, your health care provider might ask you to bend in different directions to test the range of motion in your spine. Your provider might try to reproduce your pain by pressing on specific portions of your pelvis or by moving your legs into a particular position. You also may be asked to take a deep breath to see if you have difficulty expanding your chest.

Imaging tests
X-rays allow doctors to check for changes in joints and bones, though the visible signs of ankylosing spondylitis might not be evident early in the disease.

An MRI uses radio waves and a strong magnetic field to provide more-detailed images of bones and soft tissues. MRI scans can reveal evidence of ankylosing spondylitis earlier in the disease process, but are much more expensive.

Lab tests

There are no specific lab tests to identify ankylosing spondylitis. Certain blood tests can check for markers of inflammation, but inflammation can be caused by many different health problems.

Blood can be tested for the HLA-B27 gene. But many people who have that gene don't have ankylosing spondylitis and people can have the disease without having the gene.

Treatment

The goal of treatment is to relieve pain and stiffness and prevent or delay complications and spinal deformity. Ankylosing spondylitis treatment is most successful before the disease causes irreversible damage.

Medications

Nonsteroidal anti-inflammatory drugs (NSAIDs)—such as naproxen (Aleve, Naprosyn, others) and ibuprofen (Advil, Motrin IB, others)—are the medications doctors most commonly use to treat ankylosing spondylitis. These medications can relieve inflammation, pain and stiffness, but they also might cause gastrointestinal bleeding.

If NSAIDs aren't helpful, your doctor might suggest starting a tumor **necrosis** factor (TNF) blocker or an interleukin-17 (IL-17) inhibitor. These drugs are injected under the skin or through an intravenous line. These types of medications can reactivate untreated **tuberculosis** and make you more prone to infections.

Examples of TNF blockers include:

- Adalimumab (Humira)
- **Certolizumab pegol** (Cimzia)
- **Etanercept** (Enbrel)
- Golimumab (Simponi)
- Infliximab (Remicade)

Therapy

Physical therapy is an important part of treatment and can provide a number of benefits, from pain relief to improved strength and flexibility. A physical therapist can design specific exercises for your needs. To help preserve good posture, you may be taught:

- Range-of-motion and stretching exercises
- Strengthening exercises for abdominal and back muscles
- Proper sleeping and walking positions

Surgery

Most people with ankylosing spondylitis don't need surgery. Surgery may be recommended if you have severe pain or if a hip joint is so damaged that it needs to be replaced.

Lifestyle and home remedies

Lifestyle choices can also help manage ankylosing spondylitis.

- Stay active. Exercise can help ease pain, maintain flexibility and improve your posture.
- Don't smoke. If you smoke, quit. Smoking is generally bad for your health, but it creates additional problems for people with ankylosing spondylitis, including further hampering breathing.
- Practice good posture. Practicing standing straight in front of a mirror can help you avoid some of the problems associated with ankylosing spondylitis.

(992 words)

◆ **Vocabulary**

ankylosing spondylitis [医] 强直性脊柱炎
fuse [fjuːz] *vt.* 熔化;融合
hunch[hʌntʃ] *v.* 弓身,弓背;弯腰驼背
uveitis[ˌjuːvɪˈaɪtɪs] *n.* 葡萄膜炎,眼色素层炎
crumple [ˈkrʌmp(ə)l] *vt.* 弄皱;使一蹶不

振 *vi.* 起皱
necrosis [neˈkrəʊsɪs] *n.* 坏死;坏疽;骨疽
tuberculosis [tjuːˌbɜːkjuˈləʊsɪs] *n.* 结核病
Certolizumab pegol 赛妥珠单抗
Etanercept [eɪtənəˈsept] *n.* 依那西普

附录 1　常用医学英语词缀

Ⅰ. Commonly-used medical prefix

a(n)-	without 没有	amorphous 无定型的,无组织的 anaesthesia 麻木
abdomino-	abdomen 腹部	abdominocentesis 腹部穿刺 abdominoscopy 腹腔镜检查
adeno-	gland 腺体	adenopathy 腺病 adenectomy 腺切除术
anti-	against 反…的,抗…的	antidote 解毒剂 antivirus 抗病毒的
angio-	vessel 血管	angiogram 血管造影 angioma 血管瘤
appendico-	appendix 阑尾	appendicitis 阑尾炎 appendiceal 阑尾的
arterio-	artery 动脉	arteriosclerosis 动脉硬化 arterionecrosis 动脉坏死
arthro-	joint 关节	arthritis 关节炎 arthroedema 关节水肿
atrio-	cavity, atrium 心房	atrionector 窦房结 atriotomy 心房切开术
audio-	hearing 听的	audiometer 听力计 audiphone 助听器
auto-	self 自身的	autotrophic 自给营养的 autograft 自体移植
broncho-	bronchus 支气管	bronchoadenitis 支气管淋巴结炎 bronchorrhea 支气管粘液溢
cardio-	heart 心脏	electrocardiogram 心电图 cardiogenic 心源性的
cerebro-	brain 大脑	cerebroma 脑瘤 cerebrosis 脑病
cervico-	cervix, neck 颈	cervicodynia 颈痛 cervicitis 子宫颈炎
chondro-	cartilage 软骨	chondroangioma 软骨血管瘤 chondrocyte 软骨细胞
corono-	crown 冠状部	coronary 冠状动脉的 coronoid 冠状的

cysto-	sac, bladder 膀胱	cystitis 膀胱炎
		cystoscope 膀胱镜
cyto-	cell 细胞	cytocinesis 胞质分裂
		cytoclasis 细胞破碎
dermo-	skin 皮肤	epidermis 表皮
		dermoid 皮状的,皮样的
dermato-	dermatoplasty 植皮术	dermatosis 皮肤病
		dermatology 皮肤医学,皮肤病学
duodeno-	duodenum 十二指肠	duodenectomy 十二指肠切除术
		duodenostomy 十二指肠造口术
embryo-	embryo 胚胎	embryogeny 胚胎发生
		embryoma 胎组织瘤
encephalo-	brain 大脑	encephalitis 脑炎
		encephalohemia 脑充血
entero-	intestine 肠	enterogastritis 肠胃炎
		enterogram 肠动图
epi-	over, upon, on 上,旁,表	epidermis 表皮,上皮
		epiblast 上胚层,外胚层
erythro-	red 红	erythroderma 红皮病
		erythrocyturia 红细胞尿,血尿
esophago-	esophagus 食管	esophagectomy 食管切除术
		esophagitis 食管炎
eu-	good,normal 佳,优,正常	eutocia 顺产
		eupnea 呼吸正常,平静呼吸
exo-	external 外	exocrinology 外分泌学
		exogenous 外生的,外因的
fungi-	fungus 真菌	fungicide 杀真菌剂
		fungiform 真菌状的
gastro-	stomach 胃	gastritis 胃炎
		gastroenteritis 胃肠炎
hemo-	blood 血液	hemorrhage 出血
		hemoglobin 血红蛋白
hemoto-	hematuria 血尿	hematopathy 血液病
		hemotoxic 血中毒的
hepato-	liver 肝	hepatitis 肝炎
		hepatosplenomegaly 肝脾肥大
hyper-	above, excessive 高于,超过	hypertention 高血压
		hypersensitivity 过敏
hypo-	under 在…之下	hypoglycemia 低血
		hypotention 低血压症
hystero-	uterus 子宫	hysteroptosis 子宫下垂
		hysteromyoma 子宫肌瘤
immuno-	safe, immune 免疫	immunology 免疫学

in-	not 无,不	immunoreaction 免疫反应
		inactivation 灭活
		inalimental 无营养的
intra-	within 在…内部	intravenous 静脉内的
		intracerebral 大脑内的
laryngo-	larynx 喉	laryngitis 喉炎
		laryngocele 喉囊肿
leuko-	white 白	leukorrhea 白带
		leukemia 白血病
litho-	stone, calculus 结石	lithectomy 切开取石术
		lithogenesis 结石形成
lympho-	lymph 淋巴	lymphocythemia 淋巴细胞增多症
		lymphocytoma 淋巴细胞瘤
mal-	bad 不良,坏	malnutrition 营养不良
		malabsorption 吸收不良
melano-	black 黑	melanoplakia 黑斑病
		melanosis 黑变病
meno-	menstruation 月经	menopause 绝经
		menorrhalgia 痛经
meso-	middle 中间,正中	mesoblast 中胚层
metro-	uterus 子宫	metrography 子宫照相术
		metroptosis 子宫脱垂
myelo-	spinal cord 脊髓,骨髓	myelitis 脊髓炎
		bone marrow myelocyte 髓细胞
myo-	muscle 肌肉	myocarditis 心肌炎
		myoma 肌瘤
naso-	nose 鼻子	nasopharyngitis 鼻咽炎
		nasology 鼻科学
necro-	death 坏死	necrosis 坏死
		necrocytosis 细胞坏死
nephro-	kidney 肾脏	nephritis 肾炎
		nephrectomy 肾切除术
neuro-	nerve 神经	neuroanatomy 神经解剖学
		neurology 神经学
oculo-, ophthalmo-	eye 眼	oculopathy 眼病
		oculopupillary 瞳孔的
osteo-	bone 骨	osteoblast 成骨细胞
		osteoarthropathy 骨关节病
pancreato-	pancreas 胰腺	pancreatoblastoma 胰母细胞瘤
		pancreatography 胰造影术
patho-	disease 疾病	pathogen 病原体
		pathology 病理学
parasito-	parasite 寄生虫	parasitology 寄生虫学

		parasitoid 拟寄生
peri-	around 在…周围	pericardium 心包
		pericolitis 结肠周炎
pharmaco-	medicine 药	pharmacopedia 制药学
		pharmacopeia 药典
pharyngo-	pharnx 咽	pharyngitis 咽炎
		pharyngodynia 咽痛
pneumono-	air, lung 气体，肺	pneumonia 肺炎
		pneumonorrhagia 肺出血
post-	after, behind 在…之后	postnatal 产后的
		postoperational 术后的
pre-	before 前	preoperational 术前的
		presuppurative 化脓前的
procto-	rectum 直肠	proctoplasty 直肠成形术
		proctoptosis 直肠脱垂
prostato-	prostate gland 前列腺	prostatectomy 前列腺切除术
		prostatitis 前列腺炎
pyo-	pus 脓	pyogenes 生脓的
		pyogenesis 脓生成
pulmo-	lung 肺	pulmogram 肺 X 线片
		pulmonitis 肺炎
rachio-	spinalcolumn 脊柱	rachitis 脊柱炎
		rachicentesis 椎管穿刺
reno-	kidney 肾脏	renin 肾素
		renopathy 肾病
rhino-	nose 鼻子	rhinitis 鼻炎
		rhinorrhagia 鼻出血
spermato-	semen 精液，精子	spermatoblast 精细胞，精子细胞
		spermatocyst 生精囊
spleno-	spleen 脾	splenomegaly 脾肿大
		splenitis 脾炎
stomato-	mouth 口腔	stomatodynia 口腔痛
		stomatology 口腔学
supra-	above 上，在上	supra-acromial 肩峰上的
		supra-anal 肛门上的
sympatho-	sympathetic nerve 交感神经	sympathoblast 成交感神经细胞
		sympatholytic 阻滞交感神经的
tacho-	quick 快的	tachycardia 心动过速
		tachyuria 排尿急促
thoraco-	chest 胸	thoracostenosis 胸廓狭窄
		thoracodynia 胸痛
thyro-	thyroid 甲状腺	thyroaplasia 甲状腺发育不全
		thyrocele 甲状腺肿

tonsillo-	tonsil 扁桃体	tonsillitis 扁桃体炎
		tonsillolith 扁桃体石
toxico-	poisoning 毒	toxicologist 毒理学家
		toxicosis 中毒
tracheo-	trachea 气管	tracheoaerocele 气管气疝
		tracheobronchitis 气管支气管炎
traumato-	wound 创伤	traumatology 创伤学
		traumatotherapy 创伤治疗法
typho-	typhoid 伤寒	typhosepsis 伤寒毒血症
		typhotoxin 伤寒菌毒素
uretero-	ureter 输尿管	ureterolith 输尿管结石
		ureteropyosis 输尿管化脓
urethro-	urethra 尿道	urethritis 尿道炎
		urethralgia 尿道痛
uro-	urine 尿	uremia 尿毒症
		uroclepsia 尿失禁
vagino-	vagina 阴道	vaginitis 阴道炎
		vaginodynia 阴道痛
veno-	vein 静脉	venoclysis 静脉输注
		venosclerosis 静脉硬化
viscero-	viscerus 内脏	visceroptosis 内脏下垂
		visceromegaly 内脏巨大

Ⅱ. Commonly-used medical suffixes

-ase	enzyme 酶	protease 蛋白酶
		lipase 脂肪酶
-algia	pain 疼痛	arthralgia 关节痛
		spondylalgia 脊椎痛
-blast	undifferentiated cell 未分化的细胞	hemocytoblast 原血细胞
	primitive, embryonic 胚细胞	osteoblast 成骨细胞
-cele	hernia, herniation 疝	thyrocele 甲状腺肿
		arthrocele 关节肿大
-centesis	surgical puncture 穿刺	amniocentesis 羊膜穿刺术
		celiocentesis 腹腔穿刺术
-clasia, -clasis	distuction, breaking 破坏，折断	osteoclasia 折骨术
		arthroclasia 关节活动术
-cyte	cell 细胞	leucocyte 白细胞
		erythrocyte 红细胞
-dynia	pain 痛	arthrodynia 关节痛
-ectasis, -ectasia	stretching, dilatation 扩张	bronchiolectasis 细支气管扩张
		arteriectasia 动脉扩张
-ectomy	cutting off 切除术	gastrectomy 胃切除术
		nephrectomy 肾切除术

-edema	edema 水肿	encephaledema 脑水肿
		nephredema 肾盂积水
-emesis, -ptysis	vomiting 吐	hematemesis 吐血
-emia	blood condition 血，血症	leukemia 白血病
		uremia 尿毒症
-emphraxis	obstruction 阻塞	pharyngemphraxis 咽阻塞
		laryngemphraxis 喉阻塞
-genesis	uction, development 形成，发育	hemogenesis 造血作用
		gamogenesis 有性生殖
-graph	picture, photo 图像，照片，描记仪	cardiograph 心动描计器
		photolithograph 照相平版（印刷品）
-graphy	method for writing 书写或描记的 方式、方法	electrocardiography 心电描记法
		cytography 细胞论
-hale, -spire	breathe 呼吸	inhale 吸气
		respire 呼吸
-hidrosis	sweating 汗	anhidrosis 无汗症
		polyhidrosis 多汗
-in	a chemical substance（化学物质）…素	gastrin 胃泌激素
		erythropoietin 红细胞生成素
-itis	inflammation 发炎	gastritis 胃炎
		enteritis 肠炎
-lithiasis	production of calculi 结石	cholelithiasis 胆结石
		nephrolithiasis 肾结石
-lysis	dissolution 溶解，分解	arthrolysis 关节松解术
		erythrolysis 红细胞溶解
-malacia	softening 软化	osteomalasia 骨软化
		myomalacia 肌软化
-megaly	enlargement 肿大，肥大	hepatomegaly 肝大
		splenomegaly 脾大
-meter	instrument for measuring 测量工具	thermometer 体温计
		audiometer 听力计
-metry	measurement 测量	pelvimetry 骨盆测量
		micrometry 测微法
-natal	birth 出生	postnatal 出生后，后天
		prenatal 出生前，先天
-oma	swelling, tumor 肿块，肿瘤	sarcoma 肉瘤
		angioma 血管瘤
-penia	deficiency, lack 缺乏	leucocytopenia 白细胞减少
		thrombocytopenia 血小板减少症
-pnea	breathing 呼吸	dyspnea 呼吸困难
		tachypnea 呼吸急促
-plasty	surgical repair 成形术，整形	dermatoheteroplasty 异皮移植术
		tympanoplasty 鼓膜成形术

-ptosis	falling, or the dropping 下垂	nephroptosis 肾下垂
		gastrioptosis 胃下垂
-pathy	disease; treatment 病；疗法	cardiopathy 心脏病
		hemopathy 血液病
-pexy	fixation 固定术	hysteropexy 子宫固定术
		urethropexy 尿道固定术
-orrhagia	bleeding, exudating of fluid 出血，排除液体	arthrorrhagia 关节出血
		encephalorrhagia 脑出血
-rrhaphy	suture 缝合	gastrorrhaphy 胃缝合术
		splenorrhaphy 脾缝合术
-orrhea	flow, discharge 流出，排出	hematorrhea 大出血
		pyorrhea 脓溢
-orrhexis	rupture 破裂	hepatorrhexis 肝破裂
		amniorrhexis 羊膜破裂
-sclerosis	hardening 硬化	arteriosclerosis 动脉硬化
		dermatosclerosis 硬皮病
-scope	instrumentfor viewing 镜	microscope 显微镜
		gastroscope 胃镜
-stasis	arresting, halting 阻碍，阻止	bacteriostasis 抑菌作用
		hemostasis 止血
-stenosis	a narrowing, a stricture 狭窄	arteriostenosis 动脉狭窄
		bronchostenosis 支气管狭窄
-stomy	anastomosis 造口术，吻合术	gastrostomy 胃造口术
		enterostomy 肠造口术
-therapy	treatment 疗法	chemotherapy 化学疗法
		hydrotherapy 水疗法
-tome	instrumentforcutting 刀	arthrotome 关节刀
		craniotome 开颅器
-tomy	incision 切开术	gastrotomy 胃切开术
		laparotomy 剖腹手术
-trophy, -trophia	nutrition 营养	dystrophy 营养不良
		heterotrophia 营养异常，异养性

附录 2　门诊病例常用缩略语

aa.	each	各
a.c.	before meals	饭前
aq.	water	水
B.P.	blood pressure	血压
b.i.d.	twice a day	一天两次
C.C.	chief complaint	主诉
dil.	diluted	稀释
ECG	electrocardiogram	心电图
G.C.	general condition	一般情况
H/O	history of	有…史
h.s.,hs	at bedtime	睡觉时
inj.	injection	注射
i.m.	intramuscular injection	肌肉注射
i.v.	intravenous injection	静脉注射
Imp.	impression/diagnosis	诊断
N.A.D.	nothing abnormal detected	检查无异常
O.U., o.u., ou, OU	both eyes	双眼
P.	pulse	脉搏
p.c.	after food	饭后
p.o., po, PO	orally / by mouth	口服
P.E.	physical examination	体格检查
p.r.n., prn, PRN	as needed	必要时
P.V.	per vagina	经阴道
q.4.h., q4h	every 4 hours	每 4 小时
q.d.	once a day	一天一次
q.i.d.	4 times a day	一天四次
q.o.d.	once in 2 days	隔天一次
R.	respiration	呼吸
Rp.	response/treatment	治疗
Rx	prescription	处方
s.o.s.	if necessary	需要时
T.	temperature	体温
tab.	tablet	片剂
t.i.d.	3 times a day	一天三次

附录 3　医疗卫生人员职衔职称

医学教授	professor of medicine
主任医师（医疗）	chief physician
主治医师	doctor-in-charge, visiting /attending doctor
内科主任	physician-in-chief
内科主治医师	physician-in-charge, visiting /attending physician
内科医师	physician, internist
外科主任	surgeon-in-chief
外科主治医师	surgeon-in-charge, visiting /attending surgeon
外科医师	surgeon
泌尿外科医师	urological surgeon; urologist
心脏外科医师	cardiac surgeon
胸科医师	chest physician
整形外科医师	plastic surgeon
矫形外科医师	orthopedist
妇科主治医师	gynaecologist-in-charge, visiting/attending gynaecologist
妇科医师	gynecologist
产科主治医师	obstetrician-in-charge
产科医师	obstetrician
儿科主任医师	chief physician of paediatrics
儿科医师	pediatrician
眼科主治医师	oculist-in-charge, attending oculist, visiting ophthalmologist
眼科医师	oculist; ophthalmologist
牙科主治医师	dentist-in-charge, attending/visiting dentist
牙科医师	dentist
耳鼻喉科医师	otolaryngologist
皮肤科医师	dermatologist
精神科医师	psychiatrist
传染病科医师	doctor for infectious disease
放射科医师	radiologist
理疗科医师	physiotherapist; physiotherapeutist
X线技师	X-ray technician
验光师	optometrist
麻醉师	anesthetist
全科医生	general practitioner（GP）
医师	doctor, physician
医士	assistant doctor/physician

主任护师	chief nurse
主管护师	nurse-in-charge
护师	nurse practitioner
护士	nurse
主任技师	senior technologist
主管技师	technologist-in-charge
技师	technologist
技士	technician
实习医生	intern
注册医生	registered doctor
实习护士	practice nurse
注册护士	registered nurse
护士长	head nurse
主任药师	chief pharmacist
主管药师	pharmacist-in-charge
药师	pharmacist
药士	assistant pharmacist
院长	director/superintendent of the hospital
科主任	head/chief of the department
门诊部主任	head of the out-patient department
住院部主任	head of the in-patient department
总护士长	chief head nurse
教授	professor
副教授	associate professor
讲师	lecturer
助教	assistant

附录 4 医院常见科室名称汉英对照

内科	Medical Dept., Dept.of Internal Medicine	麻醉科	Anesthesia Dept.
		放射科	Radiology Dept.
内分泌科	Endocrinology Dept.	核医学科	Nuclear Medicine Dept.
消化内科	Digestive System Dept.	针灸科	Acupuncture and Moxibustion Dept.
神经内科	Internal Neurology Dept.		
肾内科	Internal Urology Dept.	皮肤科	Dermatology Dept.
心内科	Internal Cardiology Dept.	耳鼻喉科	ENT（Ear-Nose-Throat）Dept.
心血管内科	Vasculocardiology Dept, Department of Cardiovascular Medicine	精神病科	Psychiatry Dept.
		痔疮科	Hemorrhoids Dept.
		康复科	Rehabilitation Dept.
心脏病科	Cardiology Dept.	保健科	Medical Care Dept.
血液病科	Hematology Dept.	理疗科	Physiotherapy Dept.
呼吸科	Respiration Dept.	按摩科	Massage Dept.
外科	Surgical Dept., Dept.of Surgery	临床检验科	Clinical Examination Dept.
普外科	General Surgery Dept.	传统放射科	Traditional Radiology Dept.
骨科	Orthopedics Dept.	病理科	Pathology Dept.
胸外科	Thoracic Surgery Dept.	输血科	Blood Transfusion Dept.
心外科	Cardiac Surgery Dept.	超声诊断科	Ultrasonic Diagnosis Dept.
胸心外科	Cardio-Thoracic Surgery Dept.	介入科	Intervention Dept.
神经外科	Neurological Surgery Dept.	超声多普勒室	Utrasonic Doppler Rm.
矫形外科	Orthopedic Surgery Dept.	体外反搏室	External Counterpulsation Rm.
整形外科	Plastic Surgery Dept.	化验室	Laboratory Rm.
创伤外科	Traumatology Dept.	脑电图室	ECG Rm.
泌尿外科	Urologic Surgery Dept.	胃镜室	Gastroscope Laboratory Rm.
肿瘤外科	Oncology Surgery Dept.	MR 室	MR Laboratory Rm.
小儿外科	Pediatric Surgery Dept.	SCT 室	SCT Rm.
小儿科	Pediatrics Dept.	ECT 室	ECT Rm.
儿科心理学科	Pediatric Psychology Dept.	DSA 室	DSA Rm.
泌尿科	Urology Dept.	肺功能室	Lung Function Rm.
烧伤科	Dept. of Burn	人工肾室	Hemodialyses Rm.
中医科	Traditional Chinese Medicine Dept.	血液成分分离室	Blood Composition Analysis Rm.
妇产科	Obstetric and Gynecologic Dep.	血液净化室	Blood Purification Rm.
口腔科	Stomatology Dept.	高压氧舱室	Hyperbaric Chamber
牙科	Dental Dept.	营养室	Nutrition Rm.
眼科	Ophthalmology Dept.	供应室	Supply Dept.

手术室	Operation Rm.	护理部	Nursing Dept.
候诊室	Waiting Rm.	高干病房	Senior Officials' In-patient Ward
诊室	Consulting Rm.		
急诊室	Emergency Rm.	华侨病房	Overseas Chinese Ward
医技科室	Medical Technology Rm.	院内感染监控室	Nosocomial Infection Monitory Rm.
血库	Blood Bank		
药房	Dispensary, Pharmacy	省级重点学科	Province-Level Key Subjects
挂号处	Registration Office	省级医疗领先	Province-Level Advanced
门诊部	Out-Patient Dept.	特色专业	Characteristic Specialty
住院处	Admitting Office	医院特色专科	Hospital-Level Characteristic Special Dept.
病房	Ward		

参考文献

中文参考文献

[1] 李永安,赵颖倩,徐春捷.新编高级国际医学期刊论文读写教程.西安:西安交通大学出版社,2020.

[2] 李永安.实用医学英语教程.北京:北京理工大学出版社,2010.

[3] 龚长华.实用医学英语写作教程.上海:世界图书出版公司,2014.

[4] 国林祥,武清宇.实用医学英语写作.青岛:中国海洋大学出版社,2013.

[5] 谢春晖,任雁,马军.实用医学英语写作.北京:中国人民大学出版社,2018.

英文参考文献

[1] ACL injury. mayoclinic.org. Retrieved July 25, 2021, from https://www.mayoclinic.org/diseases-conditions/acl-injury/symptoms-causes/syc-20350738

[2] Cassoobhoy, A. (2020). *Subarachnoid Hemorrhage*. Retrieved July 18, 2021, from https://www.webmd.com/stroke/subarachnoid-hemorrhage-overview

[3] Cervical spondylosis. mayoclinic. org. Retrieved July 25, 2021, from https://www.mayoclinic.org/diseases-conditions/cervical-spondylosis/symptoms-causes/syc-20370787

[4] Cunha, P. (2022). Cirrhosis (Liver). Retrieved June 8, 2022, from https://www.rxlist.com/cirrhosis/article.htm

[5] DerSarkissian, C. (2022).Understanding bone fractures—the basics. Retrieved May 8, 2022, from https://www.webmd.com/a-to-z-guides/understanding-fractures-basic-information

[6] Diabetes. mayoclinic.org. Retrieved July 22, 2021, from https://www.mayoclinic.org/diseases-conditions/diabetes/symptoms-causes/syc-20371444

[7] High blood pressure (hypertension). mayoclinic. org. Retrieved July 8, 2021, from https://www. mayoclinic. org/diseases-conditions/high-blood-pressure/symptoms-causes/syc-20373410

[8] Hyperthyroidism (overactive thyroid). mayoclinic. org. Retrieved July 20, 2021, from https://www. mayoclinic. org/diseases-conditions/hyperthyroidism/symptoms-causes/syc-20373659

[9] Khatri, M. (2021). Non-small-cell lung cancer. Retrieved July 20, 2021, from https://www.webmd.com/lung-cancer/non-small-cell-lung-cancer

[10] Pneumonia. mayoclinic.org. Retrieved July 10, 2021, from https://www.mayoclinic.org/diseases-conditions/pneumonia/symptoms-causes/syc-20354204

[11] Rheumatoid arthritis. mayoclinic. org. Retrieved July 22, 2021, from https://www.

mayoclinic.org/diseases-conditions/rheumatoid-arthritis/symptoms-causes/syc-20353648

[12] Robinson, J. (2021).Understanding Parkinson's disease—the basics. Retrieved Oct 8, 2021, from https://www.webmd.com/parkinsons-disease/guide/understanding-parkinsons-disease-basics

[13] Robinson, M. (2020). Sjogren's syndrome. Retrieved Aug 20, 2021, from https://www.webmd.com/a-to-z-guides/sjogrens-syndrome

[14] Sachdev, P. (2021). Stomach cancer. Retrieved Oct 15, 2021, from https://www.webmd.com/cancer/stomach-gastric-cancer